AF167742

Updates in Hypertension and Cardiovascular Protection

Series Editors

Giuseppe Mancia
Milano, Italy

Enrico Agabiti Rosei
Brescia, Italy

The aim of this series is to provide informative updates on both the knowledge and the clinical management of a disease that, if uncontrolled, can very seriously damage the human body and is still among the leading causes of death worldwide. Although hypertension is associated mainly with cardiovascular, endocrine, and renal disorders, it is highly relevant to a wide range of medical specialties and fields – from family medicine to physiology, genetics, and pharmacology. The topics addressed by volumes in the series *Updates in Hypertension and Cardiovascular Protection* have been selected for their broad significance and will be of interest to all who are involved with this disease, whether residents, fellows, practitioners, or researchers.

More information about this series at http://www.springer.com/series/15049

George S. Stergiou
Gianfranco Parati • Giuseppe Mancia
Editors

Home Blood Pressure Monitoring

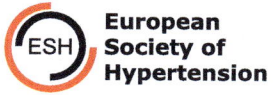

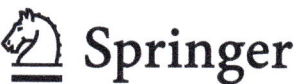

Editors
George S. Stergiou
Hypertension Center STRIDE-7
National and Kapodistrian
University of Athens
School of Medicine
Third Department of Medicine
Sotiria Hospital
Athens
Greece

Giuseppe Mancia
University of Milano-Bicocca
Milano
Italy

Gianfranco Parati
Department of Medicine and Surgery
University of Milano-Bicocca
Milano
Italy

Istituto Auxologico Italiano, IRCCS,
Department of Cardiovascular
Neural and Metabolic Sciences
Milano
Italy

ISSN 2366-4606   ISSN 2366-4614   (electronic)
Updates in Hypertension and Cardiovascular Protection
ISBN 978-3-030-23064-7   ISBN 978-3-030-23065-4   (eBook)
https://doi.org/10.1007/978-3-030-23065-4

This Springer imprint is published by the registered company Springer Nature Switzerland AG
The registered company address is: Gewerbestrasse 11, 6330 Cham, Switzerland

Preface

Self-monitoring of blood pressure at home is widely used by patients with hypertension in several countries [1]. Indeed, the clinical application of home blood pressure monitoring by patients has preceded the publication of strong research evidence from outcome studies, which are necessary to support its clinical utility in the management of hypertension [2]. Thus, despite its wide availability, scientific organizations around the world have initially hesitated to endorse the use of home blood pressure monitoring for decision-making in hypertension in clinical practice. However, in the last 20 years, the publication of several outcome studies reporting the superiority of home blood pressure monitoring compared to the conventional office measurements has now supported a major role of home monitoring in hypertension management [1–6].

Home blood pressure monitoring has unique advantages for clinical practice, particularly for repeated and long-term use, as it is widely available in most countries, is well accepted by hypertensive patients, and has relatively low cost [1, 3–6]. Thus, although ambulatory blood pressure monitoring, which is the alternative method for out-of-office blood pressure evaluation, is regarded as the gold standard method for hypertension diagnosis as it has stronger research evidence and additional unique advantages [5, 6], a pragmatic approach for most scientific societies and healthcare organizations is to promote home blood pressure monitoring as much as ambulatory monitoring, aiming to increase the number of people having their blood pressure status confirmed by out-of-office readings. When home blood pressure monitoring is applied according to the current recommendations [3–6], it can play a primary role for treatment initiation and titration in subjects with suspected or treated hypertension [7, 8]. These advantages strongly call for reimbursement of home blood pressure monitoring by healthcare systems, as done for glucose monitors in patients with diabetes [9].

The 2017 American College of Cardiology/American Heart Association guidelines for hypertension [5] and the 2018 guidelines by the European Society of Cardiology/European Society of Hypertension [6] highlighted the primary role of home blood pressure monitoring as well as of ambulatory monitoring in the diagnosis and management of hypertension. These statements on both sides of the Atlantic have started a new era in hypertension management by endorsing out-of-office blood pressure measurement as mandatory for most diagnostic and treatment decisions.

Time has come to take this method seriously [2]. As home blood pressure monitoring is already widely used, its appropriate implementation according to the current recommendations [3–6] can optimize the management of hypertension in clinical practice. This book endorsed by the European Society of Hypertension presents the current knowledge on all the aspects of home blood pressure monitoring, including the technology of devices, the clinical relevance of the method, the optimal protocol and clinical application, the clinical indications for general and special populations, the application in clinical research, and the international consensus on clinical implementation. A total of 39 international experts in blood pressure measurement research have contributed in preparing 16 chapters in this book, which aim to guide clinicians in the optimal application of home blood pressure monitoring and to stimulate researchers in filling the gaps in knowledge by performing further trials.

References

1. Stergiou GS, Kario K, Kollias A, McManus RJ, Ohkubo T, Parati G, et al. Home blood pressure monitoring in the 21st century. J Clin Hypertens. 2018;20:1116–21.
2. Stergiou GS, Siontis KC, Ioannidis JP. Home blood pressure as a cardiovascular outcome predictor: it's time to take this method seriously. Hypertension. 2010;55:1301–3.
3. Parati G, Stergiou GS, Asmar R, Bilo G, de Leeuw P, Imai Y, et al. European Society of Hypertension guidelines for blood pressure monitoring at home: a summary report of the Second International Consensus Conference on Home Blood Pressure Monitoring. J Hypertens. 2008;26:1505–26.
4. Parati G, Stergiou GS, Asmar R, Bilo G, de Leeuw P, Imai Y, et al. ESH Working Group on Blood Pressure Monitoring. European Society of Hypertension practice guidelines for home blood pressure monitoring. J Hum Hypertens. 2010;24:779–85.
5. Whelton PK, Carey RM, Aronow WS, Casey DE Jr, Collins KJ, Dennison Himmelfarb C, et al. 2017 ACC/AHA/AAPA/ABC/ACPM/AGS/APhA/ASH/ASPC/NMA/PCNA guideline for the prevention, detection, evaluation and management of high blood pressure in adults: a report of the American College of Cardiology/American Heart Association Task Force on clinical practice guidelines. Hypertension. 2018;71:e13–e115.
6. Williams B, Mancia G, Spiering W, Agabiti Rosei E, Azizi M, Burnier M, et al. ESC/ESH Guidelines for the management of arterial hypertension: The Task Force for the management of arterial hypertension of the European Society of Cardiology and the European Society of Hypertension. J Hypertens. 2018;36:1953–2041.
7. Stergiou GS, Kollias A, Zeniodi M, Karpettas N, Ntineri A. Home blood pressure monitoring: primary role in hypertension management. Curr Hypertens Rep. 2014;16:462.
8. Stergiou GS, Parati G. Home blood pressure monitoring may make office measurements obsolete. J Hypertens. 2012;30:463–5.
9. Pickering TG, Miller NH, Ogedegbe G, Krakoff LR, Artinian NT, Goff D. Call to action on use and reimbursement for home blood pressure monitoring: executive summary: a joint scientific statement from the American Heart Association, American Society of Hypertension, and Preventive Cardiovascular Nurses Association. Hypertension. 2008;52:1–9.

Contents

Devices for Home Blood Pressure Monitoring

1

Roland Asmar, Anastasios Kollias, Paolo Palatini,
Gianfranco Parati, Andrew Shennan, George S. Stergiou,
Jirar Topouchian, Ji-Guang Wang, William White,
and Eoin O'Brien

R. Asmar (✉)
Foundation-Medical Research Institutes (F-MRI®), Geneva, Switzerland
e-mail: ra@cmcv.org

A. Kollias
Hypertension Center STRIDE-7, National and Kapodistrian University of Athens,
School of Medicine, Third Department of Medicine, Sotiria Hospital, Athens, Greece

G. S. Stergiou
Hypertension Center STRIDE-7, National and Kapodistrian University of Athens, School of
Medicine, Third Department of Medicine, Sotiria Hospital, Athens, Greece
e-mail: gstergi@med.uoa.gr

P. Palatini
Department of Medicine, University of Padova, Padova, Italy
e-mail: palatini@unipd.it

G. Parati
Department of Medicine and Surgery, University of Milano-Bicocca, Milan, Italy

Istituto Auxologico Italiano, IRCCS, Department of Cardiovascular, Neural and Metabolic
Sciences, Milan, Italy
e-mail: gianfranco.parati@unimib.it

A. Shennan
Department of Women and Children's Health, School of Life Course Sciences, FoLSM,
King's College London, London, UK
e-mail: andrew.shennan@kcl.ac.uk

J. Topouchian
Diagnosis and Therapeutic Center, Hôtel Dieu Hospital, Paris, France
e-mail: jtopouchian@jtcrc.com

J.-G. Wang
The Shanghai Institute of Hypertension, Ruijin Hospital, Shanghai Jiaotong University
School of Medicine, Shanghai, China

© The Editor(s), under exclusive license to Springer Nature Switzerland AG 2020   1
G. S. Stergiou et al. (eds.), *Home Blood Pressure Monitoring*,
Updates in Hypertension and Cardiovascular Protection,
https://doi.org/10.1007/978-3-030-23065-4_1

W. White
Calhoun Cardiology Center, University of Connecticut School of Medicine, Farmington, CT, USA
e-mail: wwhite@uchc.edu

E. O'Brien
The Conway Institute, University College Dublin, Dublin, Ireland

1.1   Introduction

The use of home blood pressure (BP) monitoring (HBPM) for hypertension management is recommended by most of the international guidelines [1–4]. While these recommendations provide information on HBPM indications, procedures, and thresholds of BP values, they provide very few, or no, indications on device choice. In fact, the hypertension guidelines of the European Society of Hypertension (ESH) and the European society of cardiology (ESC) simply indicate: "HBPM …performed with semiautomatic validated BP monitors…; use of Apps as a cuff-independent means of measuring BP is not recommended; Telemonitoring and smartphone applications may offer additional advantages [4]." No other information on the device choice is indicated. The other guidelines [1–3] do not provide more indications (Table 1.1). Given the worldwide increasing dissemination of HBPM, more detailed indications on choice and use of HBPM devices are therefore necessary to guide physicians, patients, and users towards an adequate choice of suitable equipment.

In the absence of guidance on how to choose a reliable HBPM device and considering the great popularity of HBPM which is now widely available in most countries, the device market has evolved into an uncontrolled one with about 80% of marketed devices either not validated or with questionable accuracy [5]. This global BP monitoring market reached US$ 16.9 billion in 2015 and is expected to reach US$ 23.8 billion in 2020, thus being one of the most lucrative markets in the field of cardiovascular health [5, 6].

Table 1.1 Indications on HBPM devices from current hypertension guidelines

ESH/ESC	AHA/ACC	CHEP
• Semiautomatic validated BP monitor. • Memory to store and review BP data • Use of Apps as cuff-independent means of measuring BP is not recommended • Tele monitoring and smartphone Apps may offer advantages	• Use of automated validated device • BP device validated with an internationally accepted protocol • Use of auscultatory devices is not generally useful for HBPM • Monitors with data storage in memory are preferred • Use of appropriate cuff size to fit the arm	• Use only BPM devices that are appropriate for the individual and have met the standards (AAMI, ISO, BHS, ESH-IP) • Encourage devices with data recording capabilities or automatic data transmission

ESH/ESC European Guidelines [4], *AHA/ACC* American Guidelines [1], *CHEP* Canadian guidelines [3]

The widespread use of HBPM, the scientific recommendations of its use, and the large financial potential of the device market emphasize the need of device accuracy and certification and the necessity of providing clear guidance to this market by giving strict indications for the choice of HBPM devices. Publication of lists of validated home BP devices has been successfully conducted. Updated lists of the validated devices are available at several non-profit (www.bihsoc.org, https://hypertension.ca) or for-profit organizations: www.medaval.ie, www.dableducational.org [3, 7–9]. Despite the establishment of such lists, they are currently accessed only by small groups of scientists and experts and thus do not reach most of the concerned public, including physicians, pharmacists, and patients [5]. The purpose of this chapter is to describe the main characteristics of the most widely used HBPM devices and to help prescribers, consumers, and users in choosing the most reliable and suitable device.

1.2   Blood Pressure Measurement Techniques Used For HBPM

Several techniques for measuring BP are used by HBPM devices. These devices are either manual, semiautomated, or automated. Semiautomated are characterized by automatic inflation and manual cuff deflation; automated devices are characterized by automatic cuff inflation and deflation. The most widely used techniques are described below.

1.2.1   Manual Auscultatory Method

The manual auscultatory method to detect the Korotkoff sounds using either aneroid or mercury devices—where mercury manometers remain available —are not recommended for HBPM as they require substantial patient training and regular calibration [1–4].

1.2.2   Automatic Auscultatory Method

Very few devices incorporate microphones or specific sensors to perform automatic auscultatory (microphonic) measurement of BP with less user interference. Some of these devices offer automatic BP measurement using dual methods (auscultatory and/or oscillometry). Their use remains limited to exceptional cases where automatic BP measurement is problematic. Overall, the auscultatory method is not currently recommended for HBPM by clinical guidelines.

1.2.3   Oscillometric Method

Most automatic or semiautomatic electronic devices for BP measurements are using the oscillometric method [10]. Each device has its specific algorithm to calculate BP and pulse rate from the collected oscillometric signal. Most of these devices acquire data for measurements during cuff deflation whereas others do this during cuff inflation. Since each device has its own specific proprietary algorithm and technical characteristics, the measurement accuracy of one device cannot be extrapolated to another even if produced by the same manufacturer. Moreover, since the cuff in the oscillometric method is used not only to obtain arterial occlusion but also as a sensor to collect the oscillometric signal, experts agree that each oscillometric device must be used only with its own specific cuff(s) as provided by the manufacturer. Therefore, HBPM devices must be considered as the combination of a device and its accompanying cuff(s), whereas the cuff size and type used in the auscultatory method may not be applicable.

Electronic oscillometric devices require little to no training and are user-friendly, relatively inexpensive, and generally not affected by observer bias if used correctly. These devices, as well as all the other BP measurements devices, must meet the requirements of national and international regulatory bodies for medical devices such as the Food and Drug Administration (FDA) in the United States (US), and the CE (Conformité Européene) labeling according to the medical device Directives and Regulations in Europe. Since these regulations are mainly focused on safety rather than accuracy, it is recommended to use only devices that have undergone independent validation and passed the criteria of established validation protocols (CF. Accuracy).

Automatic oscillometric devices have been designed to measure BP at different arterial sites. The most popular (and recommended) ones are those measuring BP at the upper-arm (brachial artery) level and to a lesser extent those measuring BP at the wrist (radial artery) level. Even though several automated wrist devices have successfully passed recommended validation protocols, they are considered less accurate than the upper-arm devices. Oscillometric wrist device accuracy can be affected by wrist anatomy and position (with reference to the heart level), as well as by the wrist cuff characteristics (soft or pre-shaped). The pre-shaped cuffs are easier for patients to use but they conform less well than the soft one to the wrist.

Many of the electronic oscillometric devices include additional features such as memory, connectivity (PC, smartphone, or telemonitoring), and position sensor (CF Features), which may facilitate the HBPM procedures and improve its impact for hypertension management.

Taking into consideration all these aspects, current guidelines recommend the use of automated electronic oscillometric upper-arm cuff devices which meet regulatory authority requirements and have been validated according to established protocols. Moreover, some of these guidelines also do support wrist devices if used correctly in certain clinical circumstances. Indeed, wrist measurements can be helpful when the upper-arm cuff cannot be correctly fitted or is structurally impossible, such as in obese subjects with a very large upper-arm circumference.

1.2.4 Hybrid Devices

Hybrid devices have two BP measuring methods—the manual auscultatory method and the oscillometric method (CF). Even though these devices, originally developed for office BP measurement, are accurate and require less maintenance than the aneroid device, their use for HBPM is not recommended. Additionally, the use of the auscultatory method remains affected by observer bias and other disadvantages of this method; moreover, they are more expensive than most of the other digital oscillometric HBPM devices. If a hybrid device is used for HBPM, then the automatic oscillometric method would be preferable.

1.2.5 Plethysmography: Cuffless Method

For many years, many device manufacturers have been attempting to develop cuffless BP measurement devices as these would avoid many of the inconveniences associated with cuff measurements. Among these techniques such as tonometry, pulse wave velocity, pulse transit time, and plethysmography, the plethysmographic approach appears to be the most likely method to succeed [11]. Briefly, plethysmography measures volume changes. When applied to an arterial segment, the measured changes of volume are transformed into changes of pressure with calculation of systolic and diastolic BP and pulse rate values according to specific algorithms. To date, most of the cuffless devices used at the finger or at the wrist level (watches, bracelets), or even those applied at the earlobe level, are based on the plethysmographic method. These use an infrared (or other) photoelectric sensor to record changes in pulsatile blood flow by calculating the light absorption changes, which are then translated into BP values. Cuffless BP values are derived through various methods including calculation of pulse transit time, analysis of the signal using the Fast Fourier Transform (FFT) and Generalized Transfer Function (GTF), or relationships between BP and the arterial radial volume changes.

Accuracy of most plethysmography-based cuffless devices for BP measurements which may be used for HBPM remains controversial. In fact, to our knowledge, none of these very popular devices (watches, bracelets, smartphone Apps) satisfy regulatory requirements or has been validated according to currently established protocols. Therefore, despite their large distribution, mainly as multiple parameters monitoring bracelets or watches, the use of these devices is not presently recommended for HBPM as their accuracy and reliability remains highly questionable. It should be mentioned, however, that established validation standards have not been developed to assess cuffless devices and a new ISO standard for such devices is currently under development.

1.2.6 Tonometry

Principles of tonometry for measuring radial BP and performing pulse wave analysis using the transfer function has been reported and described in detail previously elsewhere [12]. Briefly, tonometry means "measuring of pressure" whereas applanation means "to flatten" the arterial wall. Applanation tonometry is performed by placing one or several tonometers (strain gauge pressure sensor) over the radial artery and applying soft pressure to obtain an assumed flattened arterial wall. This method was designed particularly for clinical use by researchers to measure the radial BP and calculate aortic (central) BP by performing the pulse wave analysis and using algorithms such as the Transfer Function. Considering the importance of aortic BP, manufacturers have tried to extrapolate the use of this technique for HBPM, but this approach is still under development and at this time remains reserved for research.

1.2.7 Other Techniques

Several other techniques to measure BP have been proposed for HBPM. The most current methods include:

- Pulse transit time: this technique is based on the assessment of pulse wave velocity and on use of its reciprocal variable, the pulse transit time, to calculate beat-by-beat BP values through a dedicated algorithm [13].
- Smartphone Apps turning the smartphone into a cuffless device. Most of these Apps use the light absorption changes from a finger to estimate changes in blood volume and to calculate finger BP values by considering the relationships between changes of blood volume and the corresponding changes in BP.

None of these techniques can be currently recommended as reliable methods for performing HBPM.

1.3 Arterial Sites: Which Are Most Suitable for HBPM?

HBPM devices measuring or calculating BP at different arterial sites are now available: upper-arm, wrist, finger, or even aortic. The choice of the arterial site is important, not only because most, if not all, of the hypertension studies have been performed using brachial BP measurements but also because BP values are not identical at the different arterial sites due to an "amplification" phenomenon.

1.3.1 Brachial Artery

Most HBPM devices measure BP at the upper-arm level (brachial artery). This measurement is currently recommended by all guidelines.

1.3.2 Radial Artery

- Oscillometric devices: several HBPM devices measuring BP at the wrist level (radial artery) are available. These devices are very popular because they are user-friendly for patients. To limit observer bias and the BP variations between brachial and radial arteries or those due to the wrist position in relation to the heart level, several wrist devices incorporate interesting features such as a position sensors or movement detectors. Some of the recently marketed wrist devices are of good quality and have passed one or more validation protocols. However, even though oscillometric wrist devices are regarded as less accurate than the upper-arm devices in daily practice, they remain useful for those conditions (e.g., severe obesity) where the upper-arm measurements may be problematic [1–4]. These recommendations are reflected in HBPM guidelines (references).

– Bracelets and Watches: several devices designed as watches or bracelets provide BP values using the photo-plethysmography method. To our knowledge, none of these devices has been validated; therefore, they cannot be recommended for HBPM.

1.3.3   Finger

Several devices or smartphone Apps provide BP values at the finger level using mainly the photo-plethysmographic method. When used to measure BP, this method can be affected by many factors which may constitute causes of error. Apart from some professional devices used in the research lab (Finapres®, Finometer® Pro), none of the other devices intended for public use has been validated. Therefore, these devices cannot be recommended for HBPM.

1.3.4   Aortic: Central BP

Considering the importance of aortic central BP and pulse wave analysis, a few HBPM devices provide central BP values and other arterial hemodynamic parameters. These values are obtained using algorithms such as a transfer function from peripheral arterial pulse waves to central pulse waves and/or other algorithms applied on the oscillometric signal recorded at the brachial artery level. Despite the importance of these parameters, their use remains reserved for research; thus, they are not recommended for routine HBPM.

1.4   Accuracy of HBPM Devices

1.4.1   Validation Protocols

Accuracy of HBPM devices is a prerequisite for correct diagnosis and management of hypertension. Thus, our task as experts and physicians should be to ensure that patients are using accurate devices and that inaccurate devices should not be made available to consumers. The quest for accuracy of BP measuring devices has been ongoing for several decades. Since the 1980s, several validation protocols have been developed. Among those most commonly used, we should mention: [1] the Association for the Advancement of Medical Instrumentation (AAMI) standard (US-based) [2, 14] the British Hypertension Society (BHS) protocol [3, 15] the European Society of Hypertension International Protocol (ESH-IP) which has been the most commonly used validation protocol during the last decade [16]; and [4] the International Organization for Standardization (ISO) standard for clinical validation of noninvasive sphygmomanometers [17]. Despite their differences, all these validation protocols have the common objective of establishing standards of accuracy for BP devices. The availability of a multitude of protocols causes confusion among physicians, users, and manufacturers but also adds difficulties in making validation a mandatory requirement. Considering these concerns, experts from ESH, AAMI, and ISO have now established a "Universal" Standard which will be applicable worldwide [18]. Therefore, experts agree that BP device validation studies must follow this single protocol, and that in the future only devices that have passed validation based on this "Universal" protocol will be used for HBPM.

1.4.2 General and Special Populations

Validation protocols include several procedures related to subject selection. Usually, subjects recruited for a validation study must represent the so-called "general population" defined as adults with no specific condition (other than hypertension) or major associated disease, and covering well-defined BP ranges, arm circumferences, and gender distribution. Since there is evidence that in several special populations automatic BP devices may have different levels of precision than in the general population, it makes sense to ask that validation of HBPM devices must be performed in both general and special populations if that is the intended future use for that device [19–21].

Special populations are defined as those with theoretical and clinical evidence that may affect accuracy of BP monitors. Experts agree that young children, pregnant women (including preeclampsia), subjects with a large arm circumference (>42 cm), and patients with arrhythmias must be considered as special populations [18]. Patients with chronic arrhythmias have been usually excluded from validation studies. Recent evidence is available that, when specifically tested in patients with arrhythmias, automated BP measurement is considered as uncertain or with reasonable accuracy [22, 23]. Other conditions which could be considered as "special populations" include adolescents, individuals aged >80 years, and those with diabetes or end-stage renal disease who have modified arterial hemodynamics. However, it is still unclear to what extent this may affect accuracy of HBPM devices. It is important to highlight that all these special populations constitute a very large part of patients attending hypertension centers. Therefore, the choice of validated HBPM devices must consider also individual phenotypes.

1.5   Cuff Issues and HBPM

Blood pressure cuff issues in HBPM are of high importance for accurate measurements; a specific chapter in this book has been dedicated to this subject. Considering that the majority of HBPM is performed using semiautomatic upper-arm devices, it is of high importance that devices be used with their specifically designed cuff(s) according to the manufacturer recommendations. Interchangeability of cuffs is strongly discouraged.

1.6   Device Features

Most HBPM devices include several features to either facilitate successful HBPM readings or to increase accuracy of BP values.

1.6.1   Blood Pressure Parameters

All automatic HBPM devices provide systolic and diastolic BP as well as the pulse rate. Some devices provide additional BP values such as mean arterial pressure or pulse pressure.

1.6.2   Other Parameters

Additional parameters can be acquired such as single lead electrocardiogram (ECG), blood glucose, oximetry, central BP, or arterial hemodynamic parameters derived from pulse wave analysis. Some devices now will calculate the shock index (heart rate/systolic blood pressure) that may be used to monitor vital signs in conditions such as hemorrhage and sepsis [24].

1.6.3   Built-in Memory

Most of the HBPM monitors include a built-in memory which allows storage and review of BP measurements for one or more users. These devices are preferred to those without such features.

1.6.4   Communication: Data Transmission

Different techniques are used to download data from the monitor: (1) wired (USB cable) or wireless connection to a computer and (2) Wi-Fi or Bluetooth connections to smartphones or tablets via specific Apps or other servers. These features are very important to enable the incorporation of HBPM data in telemedicine. Currently, these devices are preferable and used frequently in hypertension specialty centers. A chapter in this book is dedicated to these specific issues.

1.6.5   Averaging Function

Some HBPM devices can be used in mode "Average" or "Repeat" which allow repetition of 2 or 3 BP measurements at about 1-min interval and display their average with or without the first measurement. This averaging function may facilitate achieving a standardization of HBPM.

1.6.6   Position Sensor

In order to avoid positioning errors, some wrist devices have a built-in position sensor that allows BP measurement only when the wrist is in a suitable position (e.g., at the level of the heart). This function is important for limiting arm position-related errors with wrist BP devices [25].

1.6.7   Arrhythmia/Atrial Fibrillation

Most recent upper-arm or wrist HBPM devices also have a cardiac arrhythmia detection function. Some of these oscillometric devices include a specific algorithm for atrial fibrillation (AF) detection; this specific algorithm can be used also for opportunistic AF screening in the elderly according to the NICE guideline [26].

1.7   HBPM Devices: State of the Market

The market for BP measuring devices is very large and active; its financial attraction created a substantial market often driven principally by the lure of profitability. This phenomenon has resulted in a market in which about 80% of devices are either without validation or with questionable accuracy. To help providing assistance to physicians and users of HBPM lists of all validated devices have been made available by either scientific, not-for-profit or private institutions. Updated lists of validated devices are published on the internet and are available at several websites. Therefore, it would be important to check the listings of the validated HBPM devices before purchasing or prescribing them.

References

1. Whelton PK, Carey RM, Aronow WS, Casey DE Jr, Collins KJ, Dennison Himmelfarb C, et al. 2017 ACC/AHA/AAPA/ABC/ACPM/AGS/APhA/ASH/ASPC/NMA/PCNA guideline for the prevention, detection, evaluation, and management of high blood pressure in adults: a report of the American College of Cardiology/American Heart Association task force on clinical practice guidelines. Hypertension. 2018;71:e13–e115.
2. NICE: National Institute for Health and Care Excellence. Hypertension in adults: The clinical management of primary hypertension in adults. Clinical guideline 127; 2011. http://www.nice.org.uk/guidance/cg127. Accessed 11 Jan 2019.
3. Nerenberg K, Zarnke K, Leung A, Dasgupta K, Butalia S, McBrien K, et al. Hypertension Canada's 2018 guidelines for diagnosis, risk assessment, prevention, and treatment of hypertension in adults and children. Can J Cardiol. 2018;34:506–25.
4. Williams B, Mancia G, Spiering W, Agabiti Rosei E, Azizi M, Burnier M, et al. 2018 ESC/ESH guidelines for the management of arterial hypertension: the task force for the management of arterial hypertension of the European Society of Cardiology and the European Society of Hypertension. J Hypertens. 2018;36(10):1953–2041.

5. O'Brien E, Alpert B, Stergiou G. Accurate blood pressure measuring devices: influencing users in the 21st century. J Clin Hypertens. 2018;20:1138–41.
6. Research & Markets. Patient monitoring device: global markets. http://www.researchandmarkets.com/reports/3768929/-patient-monitoring-devices-global-markets#rela8. Accessed 11 Jan 2019.
7. DABL Educational Trust. Devices for blood pressure measurement. http://www.dableducational.org. Accessed 11 Jan 2019.
8. Medaval. Blood pressure monitors. https://medaval.ie/device-category/blood-pressure-monitors.
9. British and Irish Hypertension Society. www.bihsoc.org/bp-monitors/. Accessed 11 Jan 2019.
10. Alpert BS, Quinn D, Gallick D. Oscillometric blood pressure: a review for clinicians. J Am Soc Hypertens. 2014;8(12):930–8.
11. Xing X, Sun M. Optical blood pressure estimation with photo plethysmography and FFT based neural networks. Biomed Opt Express. 2016;7:3007–20.
12. Salvi P, Grillo A, Parati G. Noninvasive estimation of central blood pressure and analysis of pulse waves by applanation tonometry. Hypertens Res. 2015;38(10):646–8.
13. Bilo G, Zorzi C, Oghoa Munera JE, Torlasco C, Giuli V, Parati G. Validation of the Somnotouch™ NIBP non-invasive continuous blood pressure monitor according to the European Society of Hypertension International Protocol revision 2010. Blood Press Monit. 2015;20(5):291–4.
14. Noninvasive sphygmomanometers—part 2: clinical investigation of automated measurement type. American National Standards Institute. ANSI/AAMI/ISO 81060-2:2013. http://webstore.ansi.org. Accessed 11 Jan 2019.
15. O'Brien E, Petrie J, Littler WA, De Swiet M, Padfield PL, Altman D, et al. The British hypertension society protocol for the evaluation of blood pressure measuring devices. J Hypertens. 1993;11(Suppl 2):S43–63.
16. O'Brien E, Atkins N, Stergiou G, Karpettas N, Parati G, Asmar R, et al. Working group on blood pressure monitoring of the European Society of Hypertension. European Society of Hypertension International Protocol revision 2010 for the validation of blood pressure measuring devices in adults. Blood Press Monit. 2010;15:23–38.
17. Noninvasive sphygmomanometers: clinical validation of automated measurement type. International Organization for Standardization (ISO) 81060–2, 2009. www.iso.org. Accessed 11 Jan 2019.
18. Stergiou G, Alpert B, Mieke S, Asmar R, Atkins N, Eckert S, et al. A universal standard for the validation of blood pressure measuring devices: Association for the Advancement of Medical Instrumentation/European Society of Hypertension/International Organization for Standardization (AAMI/ESH/ISO) Collaboration Statement. J Hypertens. 2018;36:472–8.
19. Azaki A, Diab R, Harb A, Asmar R, Chahine MN. Questionable accuracy of home blood pressure measurements in the obese population—validation of the microlife WatchBP O3® and Omron RS6® devices according to the European Society of Hypertension-International Protocol. Vasc Health Risk Manag. 2017;2(13):61–9.
20. Padwal RS, Majumdar SR. Comparability of two commonly used automated office blood pressure devices in the severely obese. Blood Press Monit. 2016;21(5):313–5.
21. Stergiou GS, Asmar R, Myers M, Palatini P, Parati G, Shennan A, et al. European Society of Hypertension Working Group on Blood Pressure Monitoring and Cardiovascular Variability. Improving the accuracy of blood pressure measurement: the influence of the European Society of Hypertension International Protocol (ESH-IP) for the validation of blood pressure measuring devices and future perspectives. J Hypertens. 2018;36(3):479–87.
22. Stergiou GS, Dolan E, Kollias A, Poulter NR, Shennan A, Staessen JA, et al. Blood pressure measurement in special populations and circumstances. J Clin Hypertens (Greenwich). 2018;20(7):1122–7.
23. Stergiou GS, Kollias A, Destounis A, Tzamouranis D. Automated blood pressure measurement in atrial fibrillation: a systematic review and meta-analysis. J Hypertens. 2012;30(11):2074–82.

24. Nathan H, Vousden N, Lawley E, de Greeff A, Hezelgrave N, Sloan N, et al. Development and evaluation of a novel vital signs alert device for use in pregnancy in low-resource settings. BMJ Innov. 2018;0:1–7.
25. Deutsch C, Krüger R, Saito K, Yamashita S, Sawanoi Y, Beime B, et al. Comparison of the Omron RS6 wrist blood pressure monitor with the positioning sensor on or off with a standard mercury sphygmomanometer. Blood Press Monit. 2014;19(5):306–13.
26. National Institute for Health and Care Excellence 2013. Watch BP Home A for opportunistically detecting atrial fibrillation during diagnosis and monitoring of hypertension. https://www.nice.org.uk/guidance/MTG13. Accessed 11 Jan 2019.

Cuff Design for Home Blood Pressure Monitors

2

Paolo Palatini, Roland Asmar, Grzegorz Bilo, and Gianfranco Parati

2.1 Introduction

Home blood pressure (BP) measurement has a stronger predictive power for cardiovascular disease and mortality than does office BP and is recommended as a routine monitoring tool in hypertension [1]. However, self BP measurement if not properly performed may be the source of erroneous BP readings and requires the use of a reliable device and of an appropriate cuff. With the auscultatory method, the role of the cuff is to compress the artery under defined reference pressures, whereas with oscillometric devices, which are currently used for self BP measurement, the cuff is at the same time the signal sensor [2, 3]. This stresses the importance of the varying software-cuff combinations in the different measurement methods. Complete artery

P. Palatini (✉)
Department of Medicine, University of Padova, Padova, Italy
e-mail: palatini@unipd.it

R. Asmar
Foundation-Medical Research Institutes (F-MRI®), Geneva, Switzerland
e-mail: ra@cmcv.org

G. Bilo
Department of Cardiovascular Neural and Metabolic Sciences, Istituto Auxologico Italiano, IRCCS, Milan, Italy

Department of Medicine and Surgery, University of Milano-Bicocca, Milan, Italy
e-mail: g.bilo@auxologico.it

G. Parati
Department of Medicine and Surgery, University of Milano-Bicocca, Milan, Italy

Istituto Auxologico Italiano, IRCCS, Department of Cardiovascular, Neural and Metabolic Sciences, Milan, Italy
e-mail: gianfranco.parati@unimib.it

occlusion is not critical when BP is measured with the oscillometric method because oscillations can be detected also beyond the systolic pressure through the knocking of the pulse at the over inflated bladder wall [2, 3].

The characteristics of the cuff for accurate BP measurement have been the subject of much debate in the literature and many problems still remain controversial [2, 4, 5]. With traditional sphygmomanometry miscuffing is a serious source of measurement error. Use of too narrow or too short bladders (undercuffing) leads to overestimation of BP, a problem often overlooked by many doctors when measuring BP in patients with large arms. Conversely, use of too wide or too long bladders (overcuffing) may lead to BP underestimation. Moreover, when too short bladders are used, BP overestimation error may further increase whenever the bladder is not correctly centered over the course of the brachial artery. This additional bias is about 5 mmHg for systolic and 4 mmHg for diastolic BP in case of major cuff misplacement [6]. The Scientific Societies addressed the issue of miscuffing extensively but recommendations were often inconsistent (Fig. 2.1). For example, the British Hypertension Society recommends a standard cuff with a bladder measuring 12 x 26 cm for the majority of adult arms, a large cuff with a bladder measuring 12 x 40 cm for obese arms, and a small cuff with a bladder measuring 12 x 18 cm for lean adult arms and children [5]. The American Heart Association recommends the use of a totally different set of cuffs: a small adult cuff (10×24 cm) for arm circumference 22–26 cm, an adult cuff (13×30 cm) for arm circumference 27–34 cm, a large adult cuff (16×38 cm) for arm circumference 35–44 cm, and an adult thigh cuff (20×42 cm) for arm circumference 45–52 cm [7]. The European Society of Hypertension/European Society of Cardiology guidelines provide less detailed recommendations saying that a standard bladder cuff (12–13 cm wide and 35 cm long) should be used for most patients, but larger and smaller cuffs should be available for larger (arm circumference > 32 cm) and thinner arms, respectively [8].

These inconsistencies may be ascribed to the lack of a gold standard for BP measurement because of the difficulty of obtaining comparative data from intraarterial studies. At any rate, current recommendations of Scientific Bodies may not apply to oscillometric BP measurement in which the cuff is also a signal sensor. With

Fig. 2.1 Recommendations of the American Heart Association (AHA) [6], British Hypertension Society (BHS) [5], and European Society of Hypertension/European Society of Cardiology (ESH) [7] for blood pressure cuff sizes for mercury sphygmomanometers and automatic home blood pressure monitors

	Indication	Width x length (cm)	Circumference (cm)
AHA	Small adult	12 x 22	22 - 26
	Adult	16 x 30	27 - 34
	Large adult	16 x 36	35 - 44
	Adult thigh	16 x 42	45 - 52
BHS	Small adult/child	12 x 18	< 23
	Standard adult	12 x 26	< 33
	Large adult	12 x 40	< 50
	Adult thigh cuff	20 x 42	< 53
ESH	Thin arms	Small cuff	Small
	Standard adult	12-13 x 35	< 32
	Larger arms	Large cuff	≥ 32

oscillometric devices the choice of the appropriate cuff appears even more controversial because the oscillometric measurement is generated by a different sequence of events compared to the auscultatory one. One limitation of the oscillometric technique is that the oscillogram has a certain amount of variability and inconsistency in terms of asymmetry and nonuniformity of the pulsations. Thus, to eliminate potential errors in derived values of systolic and diastolic BPs innovative techniques are being continually sought that might improve the reliability of oscillometric BP measurement. A potential improvement on the existing techniques was reported some years ago by Fujikawa et al. who used a triple cuff sphygmomanometer and the pulse delay time method [9]. Although this technique provided adequate and accurate BP measurements and has the potential to be a standard tool for indirect BP measurement, it did not reach any significant application in daily practice [10].

2.2 The Bladder Size

A generally accepted rule of thumb is that for accurate BP measurements the rubber bladder inside the cuff should encircle at least 80% of the upper arm and have a width of at least 40% of the arm circumference [7]. However, an intraarterial study in which multiple indirect measurements were made using a cuff width:arm circumference ratio varying from 30% to 55% showed that optimal bladder dimensions for achieving accurate BP measurements differ from those currently recommended [11]. A ratio of 40% resulted in overestimation of BP for most arms with particularly high errors for small arms. The ratio producing zero error for the pooled study group was 46.4%. However, using the fixed 46.4% ratio the error varied inversely with arm circumference, resulting in overestimation of systolic BP for small arms and underestimation of systolic BP for large arms [11]. The optimum ratio was found to be proportional to the logarithm of the arm's circumference. These data indicate that the choice of the optimal cuff for BP measurement with the auscultatory method remains a clinical dilemma. The more so if one considers that current recommendations for cuff size may not apply to devices based on the oscillometric method. As mentioned above, complete artery occlusion is not critical when BP is measured with the oscillometric method [2, 3]. Interesting results on the biomechanical basis of oscillometric BP were provided by Han et al. using an arm model consisting of three separate cylindrical parts: soft tissue, bone, and brachial artery [12]. The artery volume changes under the cuff were used to represent the cuff pressure oscillations for analyzing BP measurements. This study showed that the measured cuff pressure oscillations are a reflection of the entire artery volume change under the cuff, thereby presenting a mixture of arterial distension in different closure states during the entire measurement process. Although the oscillation amplitude was smaller with stiff than with elastic arteries, the stiffness variation of the brachial artery did not affect the accuracy of oscillometric BP measurement. This is due to the fact that the oscillometric technique is based on the location and not on the amplitude of the oscillations. Maximum oscillations occur at the same point with any type of arterial wall, and thus the accuracy of the oscillometric BP measurement is not affected by the arterial wall characteristics. This represents an advantage of the oscillometric over the auscultatory measurement because with the latter method the cuff pressure transmission is affected by brachial artery elasticity which may lead to an overestimation of auscultatory BP up to 5% with stiff arteries and to an underestimation up to 5% with elastic arteries [12].

2.3   How to Measure BP in the Obese

As mentioned above, for an accurate BP measurement the size of the rubber bladder inside the cuff should be proportional to the circumference of the arm [13]. Thus, obese subjects will often require the use of large-sized cuffs (Fig. 2.2). However, a large arm often cannot be correctly cuffed especially in obese women with short humerus length. An arm length < 20 cm could be found in up to 22% of the subjects referred to an outpatient clinic [14]. According to the AHA recommendations, in subject with arm circumferences from 45 to 52 cm and short upper arm length, a 16 cm wide cuff can be used [7]. However, this recommendation does not satisfy the 40% arm circumference criterion and in these subjects BP measurement at the upper arm may provide inaccurate readings.

Another problem often overlooked by clinicians is that the choice of the appropriate cuff in obese individuals also depends on the upper arm shape which in the obese is tronco-conical [14, 15]. A conically shaped arm makes it difficult to fit

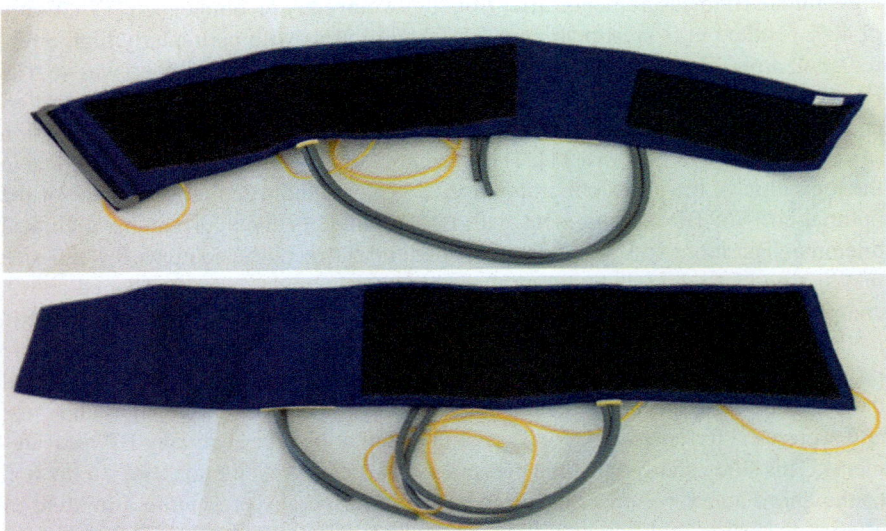

Fig. 2.2 Conical (upper part) and cylindrical (lower part) cuffs for blood pressure measurement in obese subjects with upper arm circumference at the midpoint ≥42 cm. The conical cuff is formed with upper and lower arcuate edges and is provided with a bladder having proximal and distal length of 45 and 35 cm, respectively. The slant angle of the frustum of the cone corresponding to the cuff and bladder when the cuff is encompassing a limb is 85.0°. In the cylindrical cuff, the upper and lower sides of the bladder have the same length (40 cm). For both the conical and the cylindrical cuffs the length and width are 40 and 20 cm, respectively, on the center

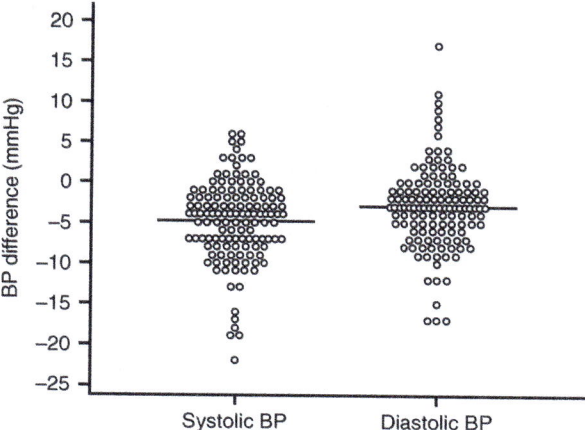

Fig. 2.3 Systolic and diastolic blood pressure differences between measurements performed with a cylindrical cuff and a tronco-conical cuff in a group of subjects ($N = 33$) with middle arm circumference $\geq$42 cm. Three blood pressure readings were obtained in each subject. The solid line indicates the mean value for the group. A negative value indicates that the cylindrical cuff measurement is greater than the tronco-conical cuff measurement. Adapted from Palatini P et al., J Hypertens 2018; Jun 20. [Epub ahead of print]

a cylindrical cuff to the arm, increasing the likelihood of inaccurate BP measurements [14]. In the past, this issue has been disregarded even by Scientific Bodies and the recent AAMI/ESH/ISO guidelines admit that there is a need for future investigations in this field [16]. It should be born in mind that the shape of the upper arm is tronco-conical in almost all individuals and that the conicity increases with increasing circumference of the arm [11]. In one study, the difference between the proximal and distal circumference of the upper arm ranged from 1 to 20 cm, with an average value of 8.7 cm [14] corresponding to slant angles ranging from 89.2° to 82.4°. A conically shaped arm prevents accurate BP measurement if a cylindrical cuff is used, because the distal part of the cuff will remain loose and will expand irregularly over the lower part of the arm during inflation causing an overestimation of the true BP [14]. A recent study [17] showed that the measurement error with a cylindrical cuff is particularly important in subjects with morbid obesity and arm circumference of 42 cm or larger. The mean BP overestimation using the cylindrical cuff was 5/3 mmHg with between-cuff differences as high as >20 mmHg (Fig. 2.3). The same problem may be encountered when a cylindrical wide-range cuff is used (see below).

2.4   The Advent of the Wide-Range Cuff

The one-size-fits-all cuff, currently called wide-range cuff, has been designed for self BP measurement at home and appeared on the market over a decade ago [18, 19]. Despite being provided with cuffs and bladders of standard size, these cuffs are claimed to yield accurate BP readings over a wide range of arm circumferences, usually from 22 to 42 cm. They can overcome the problem of miscuffing in obese individuals with short upper arm and eliminate the need to supply several different cuffs in relation to arm circumference. Indeed, these cuffs have been shown to provide accurate BP measurements over a wide range of arm sizes thanks to a special software algorithm which adjusts the device parameters based on the characteristics of the individual arm being tested [2, 18]. The specific cuff design provides stable arterial occlusion and assessment of the oscillometric signal efficiency through electronic gain adjustment in each measurement. One study showed that a single cuff with a 14.5 × 32 cm bladder could provide accurate BP readings in subjects with arm circumferences up to 50 cm [20]. As of today, 25 validation studies have been published reporting data on 28 devices coupled to a wide-range cuff [21]. However, a recent review of published validation studies indicates deficiencies in the assessment of the accuracy of wide-range cuffs [21]. One main concern was that the full range of arm circumferences was evaluated in less than 10% of the studies with the upper and lower extremes of the range being not fully assessed. This limitation was particularly relevant in validation studies performed according to the ESH-IP 2010 protocol which does not include arm size distribution among the criteria for subject recruitment [22]. In addition, it should be noted that a tronco-conical shape should be adopted also for wide-range cuffs. Indeed, one study showed that when a cylindrical wide-range cuff was used in obese subjects it consistently overestimated systolic BP, whereas when a tronco-conical cuff was used accurate BP readings could be obtained [23]. Combining tronco-conical cuff shape with improvements in the cuff internal structure, aimed at providing more homogeneous distribution of applied pressure all over the covered surface, might further improve the accuracy of oscillometric measurements in individuals with large arms [6].

2.5   Other Options for Self BP Measurement in the Obese

The use of wrist monitors may be a valid alternative for BP measurement in obese subjects especially if devices coupled to conical cuffs are used [24]. Wrist monitors may be of help especially in subjects with short upper arm [25]. Many validated wrist devices have appeared on the market in the last few decades with the advantage of being smaller and easier to use than upper arm monitors. However, in spite of technical improvement several concerns are still being raised about their reliability in real-life conditions because the accuracy of BP measurement at the wrist largely depends on the difference in height between the wrist and the heart. A recent study showed that the accuracy of BP measured at the wrist varied according to whether BP was measured in the office under doctor's supervision or at home in a real-life situation [26]. Reliable BP readings at the wrist were obtained only when BP was taken in the office, whereas when BP was self-measured at home BP measurements were inaccurate. A better alternative for the obese may be the use of devices that measure BP at the forearm although experience is still limited. As in the obese also the forearm has a conical shape, manufacturers have designed conically shaped cuffs for forearm monitors [27]. In a group of subjects whose forearm proximal and distal circumferences were 30 cm and 18 cm, respectively, a forearm device was validated against the intraarterial measurement using a tronco-conical cuff [27]. This instrumentation provided reliable BP readings across a wide range of forearm circumferences.

2.6   Arm and Cuff Size in Validation Studies

To avoid the use of unreliable BP devices several international bodies have developed protocols for the validation of BP monitors. A large number of automatic or semiautomatic devices have been validated [28] mostly using the British Hypertension Society or the ESH-IP protocol [22]. However, as mentioned above arm size is not included among the criteria used for selecting the subjects recruited for the validations performed with these protocols. The introduction of wide-range cuffs into the market has made it clear that the accuracy of these cuffs should be tested on an adequate number of subjects with arm width at both extremes of the declared arm size range. To fill this gap, the latest AAMI/ISO81060-2 protocol specified that for a sphygmomanometer intended for use with a single cuff size, at least 40% of the subjects must have a limb circumference which lies within the upper half of the specified range of use of the cuff and at least 40% must have a limb circumference within the lower half [29]. In addition, at least 20% of the subjects should have a limb circumference which lies within the upper quarter of the specified range of use of the cuff and at least 20% should have a limb circumference within the lower quarter. For a sphygmomanometer intended for use with multiple cuff sizes, each cuff size shall be tested on at least $1/(2 \times n)$ of the subjects, where n is the number of cuff sizes. These recommendations have been recently confirmed by a scientific body including AAMI, ESH, and ISO experts who developed a universal standard for device validation which is expected to replace all previous protocols [16].

2.7   Conclusions and Future Perspectives

Devices for self BP measurement at home should be provided with cuffs of optimal size and shape in relation to the patient's arm circumference. Especially when semi-rigid cuffs are used in large arms the shape of the cuff should be tronco-conical. The optimal shape of these cuffs in relation to arm size is still unclear and should be established on the basis of measurements obtained in a large number of subjects over a wide range of arm circumferences. Cylindrical and conical cuffs and bladders of different size should be constructed and compared in the various arm size classes studying the influence of sex, age, and arm adiposity. The advent of wide-range cuffs coupled to oscillometric devices has opened a new era for BP measurement in the very obese. However, although they are very promising these cuffs should be tested in larger populations over the full range of arm sizes following the requirements of the AAMI/ESH/ISO protocol.

The present BP measuring techniques are still based on cuff occlusion. However, for the reasons delineated above the cuffing technique is often difficult to apply in subjects with big arms. This problem can be overcome with the use of noninvasive cuffless BP measurement devices that measure BP using completely different techniques such as the pulse wave propagation time, from finger plethysmography, by ultrasonic sonar through a wristwatch ultrasound device, and even from a steering wheel sensor system while driving [30, 31]. The biometric information can be then transmitted to a smartphone or tablet [32]. The IEEE published a standard for wearable cuffless BP measuring devices, which was certified as IEEE1708 on 26 August 2014 [33]. The development of cuffless monitors has been thriving in the last few years and the number of patents has been increasing with over 70 registered in 2016 [30, 31]. However, the reliability of cuffless devices is still under scrutiny, and there is insufficient evidence to recommend these devices to patients at present. Collaboration between researchers, manufacturers, and clinicians will be crucial to moving these innovative techniques forward prior to incorporating them into clinical practice.

References

1. Parati G, Stergiou GS, Asmar R, Bilo G, de Leeuw P, Imai Y, Kario K, Lurbe E, Manolis A, Mengden T, O'Brien E, Ohkubo T, Padfield P, Palatini P, Pickering TG, Redon J, Revera M, Ruilope LM, Shennan A, Staessen JA, Tisler A, Waeber B, Zanchetti A, Mancia G, ESH Working Group on Blood Pressure Monitoring. European Society of Hypertension practice guidelines for home blood pressure monitoring. J Hum Hypertens. 2010;24(12):779–85.
2. Palatini P, Frick GN. Cuff and bladder: overlooked components of BP measurement devices in the modern era? Am J Hypertens. 2012;25:136–8.
3. Geddes LA, Voelz M, Combs C, Reiner D, Babbs CF. Characterization of the oscillometric method for measuring indirect blood pressure. Ann Biomed Eng. 1982;10:271–80.
4. O'Brien E. A century of confusion: which bladder for accurate blood pressure measurement? [review]. J Hum Hypertens. 1996;10:565–72.
5. O'Brien E, Petrie J, Littler WA, De Swiet M, Padfield PD, Dillon MJ. Blood pressure measurement: recommendations of the Britishn hypertension society, 3rd edn. London: BMJ Publishing Group; 1997.
6. Bilo G, Sala O, Perego C, Faini A, Gao L, Głuszewska A, Ochoa JE, Pellegrini D, Lonati LM, Parati G. Impact of cuff positioning on blood pressure measurement accuracy: may a specially designed cuff make a difference? Hypertens Res. 2017;40(6):573–80.
7. Pickering TG, Hall JE, Appel LJ, Falkner BE, Graves J, Hill MN, Jones DW, Kurtz T, Sheps SG, Roccella EJ. Recommendations for blood pressure measurement in humans and experimental animals: part 1: blood pressure measurement in humans: a statement for professionals from the Subcommittee of Professional and Public Education of the American Heart Association Council on high blood pressure research. Circulation. 2005;111:697–716.
8. Williams B, Mancia G, Spiering W, Agabiti Rosei E, Azizi M, Burnier M, Clement DL, Coca A, de Simone G, Dominiczak A, Kahan T, Mahfoud F, Redon J, Ruilope L, Zanchetti A, Kerins M, Kjeldsen SE, Kreutz R, Laurent S, Lip GYH, McManus R, Narkiewicz K, Ruschitzka F, Schmieder RE, Shlyakhto E, Tsioufis C, Aboyans V, Desormais I, Authors/Task Force Members. ESC/ESH guidelines for the management of arterial hypertension: the task force for the management of arterial hypertension of the European Society of Cardiology and the European Society of Hypertension: the task force for the management of arterial hypertension

of the European Society of Cardiology and the European Society of Hypertension. J Hypertens. 2018;36(10):1953–2041.

9. Fujikawa T, Tochikubo O, Sugano T, Umemura S. Accuracy of the pulse delay time technique with triple cuff for objective indirect blood pressure measurement. J Hypertens. 2013;31(2):278–86.

10. Parati G, Avolio A. Improvements on cuff measurement of arterial pressure: more cuffs! J Hypertens. 2013;31(2):251–2.

11. Marks LA, Groch A. Optimizing cuff width for noninvasive measurement of blood pressure. Blood Press Monit. 2000;5:153–8.

12. Lan H, Al-Jumaily AM, Lowe A, Hing W. Effect of tissue mechanical properties on cuff-based blood pressure measurements. Med Eng Phys. 2011;33:1287–92.

13. Palatini P, Parati G. Blood pressure measurement in very obese patients: a challenging problem. J Hypertens. 2011;29:425–9.

14. Palatini P, Benetti E, Fania C, Malipiero G, Saladini F. Rectangular cuffs may overestimate blood pressure in individuals with large conical arms. J Hypertens. 2012;30:530–650.

15. Maxwell GF, Pruijt JF, Arntzenius AC. Comparison of the conical cuff and the standard rectangular cuffs. Int J Epidemiol. 1985;14:468–72.

16. Stergiou GS, Alpert B, Mieke S, Asmar R, Atkins N, Eckert S, Frick G, Friedman B, Graßl T, Ichikawa T, Ioannidis JP, Lacy P, McManus R, Murray A, Myers M, Palatini P, Parati G, Quinn D, Sarkis J, Shennan A, Usuda T, Wang J, Wu CO, O'Brien E. A universal standard for the validation of blood pressure measuring devices: Association for the Advancement of medical instrumentation/European Society of Hypertension/International Organization for Standardization (AAMI/ESH/ISO) collaboration statement. Hypertension. 2018;71(3):368–74.

17. Palatini P, Benetti E, Fania C, Saladini F. Only troncoconical cuffs can provide accurate blood pressure measurements in people with severe obesity. J Hypertens. 2019;37(1):37–41.

18. Palatini P, Asmar R. Cuff challenges in blood pressure measurement. J Clin Hypertens. 2018;20(7):1100–3.

19. Stergiou GS, Tzamouranis D, Nasothimiou EG, Protogerou AD. Can an electronic device with a single cuff be accurate in a wide range of arm size? Validation of the Visomat comfort 20/40 device for home blood pressure monitoring. J Hum Hypertens. 2008;22:796–800.

20. Masiero S, Saladini F, Benetti E, Palatini P. Accuracy of the microlife large-extra large-sized cuff (32-52 cm) coupled to an automatic oscillometric device. Blood Press Monit. 2011;16:99–102.

21. Sprague E, Padwal RS. Adequacy of validation of wide-range cuffs used with home blood pressure monitors: a systematic review. Blood Press Monit. 2018;23(5):219–24.

22. O'Brien E, Atkins N, Stergiou G, Karpettas N, Parati G, Asmar R, on behalf of the Working Group on Blood Pressure Monitoring of the European Society of Hypertension. European Society of Hypertension International Protocol revision 2010 for the validation of blood pressure measuring devices in adults. Blood Press Monit. 2010;15:23–38.

23. Bonso E, Saladini F, Zanier A, Benetti E, Dorigatti F, Palatini P. Accuracy of a single rigid conical cuff with standard-size bladder coupled to an automatic oscillometric device over a wide range of arm circumferences. Hypertens Res. 2010;33(11):1186–91.

24. Parati G, Asmar R, Stergiou GS. Self blood pressure monitoring at home by wrist devices: a reliable approach? J Hypertens. 2002;20(4):573–8.

25. O'Brien E. What to do when faced with an unmeasurable ambulatory blood pressure? J Hypertens. 2011;29:451–3.

26. Casiglia E, Tikhonoff V, Albertini F, Palatini P. Poor reliability of wrist blood pressure self-measurement at home: a population-based study. Hypertension. 2016;68(4):896–903.

27. Hersh LT, Sesing JC, Luczyk WJ, Friedman BA, Zhou S, Batchelder PB. Validation of a conical cuff on the forearm for estimating radial artery blood pressure. Blood Press Monit. 2014;19:38–45.

28. Stergiou GS, Asmar R, Myers M, Palatini P, Parati G, Shennan A, Wang J, O'Brien E. Improving the accuracy of blood pressure measurement: the influence of the European

Society of Hypertension International Protocol (ESH-IP) for the validation of blood pressure measuring devices and future perspectives. J Hypertens. 2018;36:479–87.

29. Non-invasive sphygmomanometers Part 2: Clinical investigation of automated measurement type. https://www.iso.org/home.html. Accessed 21 Oct 2018.

30. Arakawa T. Recent research and developing trends of wearable sensors for detecting blood pressure. Sensors. 2018;18(9):pii: E2772.

31. Goldberg EM, Levy PD. New approaches to evaluating and monitoring blood pressure. Curr Hypertens Rep. 2016;18(6):49–56.

32. Plante TB, Urrea B, MacFarlane ZT, Blumenthal RS, Miller ER 3rd, Appel LJ, Martin SS. Validation of the instant blood pressure smartphone app. JAMA Intern Med. 2016;176(5):700–2.

33. IEEE 1708–2014—IEEE Standard for Wearable Cuffless Blood Pressure Measuring Devices. https://standards.ieee.org/standard/1708-2014.html. Accessed 21 Oct 2018.

Home Blood Pressure and Preclinical Organ Damage

3

Takayoshi Ohkubo, Kazuomi Kario, Teemu J. Niiranen, Daichi Shimbo, and Giuseppe Mancia

3.1   Introduction

Preclinical organ damage is recognized as an intermediate stage in the continuum of cardiovascular disease and a determinant of total cardiovascular risk in hypertension. Elevated blood pressure (BP) is a powerful, independent risk factor for incident

T. Ohkubo (✉)
Department of Hygiene and Public Health, Teikyo University School of Medicine, Tokyo, Japan

Tohoku Institute for Management of Blood Pressure, Sendai, Japan
e-mail: tohkubo@med.teikyo-u.ac.jp

K. Kario
Division of Cardiovascular Medicine, Department of Medicine, Jichi Medical University School of Medicine (JMU), Tochigi, Japan
e-mail: kkario@jichi.ac.jp

T. J. Niiranen
Department of Public Health Solutions, National Institute for Health and Welfare, Turku, Finland

Department of Medicine, Turku University Hospital and University of Turku, Turku, Finland
e-mail: teemu.niiranen@thl.fi

D. Shimbo
Department of Medicine, Columbia University Medical Center, New York, NY, USA
e-mail: ds2231@cumc.columbia.edu

G. Mancia
University of Milano-Bicocca, Milan, Italy
e-mail: giuseppe.mancia@unimib.it

© The Editor(s), under exclusive license to Springer Nature Switzerland AG 2020
G. S. Stergiou et al. (eds.), *Home Blood Pressure Monitoring*,
Updates in Hypertension and Cardiovascular Protection,
https://doi.org/10.1007/978-3-030-23065-4_3

23

cardiovascular diseases. Recent international hypertension management guidelines have conferred increasing weight upon home BP measurements [1, 2]. Thus, the association between home BP and preclinical organ damage is important to evaluate.

This chapter reviewed published evidence supporting an association between home BP values and preclinical organ damage.

3.2 Comparison of Strength of Association with Preclinical Organ Damage Between Home and Office BP

3.2.1 Left Ventricular Hypertrophy (LVH)

A systematic review identified a more powerful association between LVH and home BP than office BP [3]. That review evaluated ten studies that included 1832 and 1597 individuals in whom systolic and diastolic BP could be measured and assessed correlations between echocardiographic left ventricular mass index (LVMI) and home and office BP. They reported significantly higher pooled coefficients for home ($r = 0.46$ vs. 0.28 $P < 0.001$), than for office systolic/diastolic BP ($r = 0.23$ vs. 0.19, $P = 0.009$).

Several studies later confirmed closer associations between LVMI and home BP rather than office BP [4–7]. A longitudinal study also confirmed the superiority of home BP over office BP in an 11-year follow-up of LVH assessed by electrocardiography (ECG-LVH) in a sample of 615 community-dwelling participants in the Finn-Home study [8].

The interventional Study on Ambulatory Monitoring of Blood Pressure and Lisinopril Evaluation (SAMPLE) also supported the superiority of home BP over office BP [9]. The SAMPLE study examined the ability of antihypertensive treatment to reduce BP within 1 year relative to LVMI regression in 206 patients with essential hypertension and LVH. The study found that a reduction in home BP correlated slightly better with treatment-induced changes in LVMI than a reduction in office BP.

3.2.2 Carotid Atherosclerosis

A systematic review of correlations between carotid intima-media thickness (IMT) with home and office BP in pooled studies of 1222 individuals [10–13] found no significant difference in pooled r coefficients between home and office systolic/diastolic BP (home: $r = 0.25$ [95% CI, 0.07–0.41]/0.07 [95% CI, −0.20–0.32], $P = 0.48$; office: $r = 0.22$ [95% CI, 0.17–0.28]/0.07 [95% CI, −0.01–0.14], $P = 0.54$).

In contrast, two other studies found a closer association between carotid atherosclerosis and home BP than office BP. The Ohasama study by Hara et al. examined 583 individuals in a general population [14]. They defined carotid atherosclerosis as carotid mean IMT measuring >0.9 mm or findings of focal carotid plaque. They reported that adjusted odds ratios (OR) for risk of carotid atherosclerosis per 1 SD increase in each systolic BP component was significantly higher for home, than for office BP (54% [95% CI, 23% to 92%] vs. 15% ([95% CI, −5% to 39%). Matsui et al. examined 356 patients at a local hospital with hypertension that had never been treated [4]. The likelihood ratio test indicated that the goodness-of-fit of a model to predict carotid atherosclerosis was significantly improved when mean home systolic BP was added to the model based on mean office systolic BP ($P = 0.002$).

3.2.3 Urinary Protein Excretion

A systematic review including two pooled studies of 156 individuals investigated associations between urinary protein excretion and home and office BP values [10, 15]. They found that pooled r (95% CI) did not significantly differ between home and office systolic/diastolic BP (0.26 [0.10–0.40]/0.17 [−0.003–0.33], $P = 0.68$; vs. 0.21 [0.05–0.36]/0.23 [0.07–0.371], $P = 0.59$). Gaborieau et al. [11] investigated correlations between the urinary albumin/creatinine ratio (UACR) and home and office BP in 302 individuals. They also found no difference in correlations between the UACR and home and office systolic BP ($r = 0.16$ vs. 0.18).

In contrast, three other studies identified a closer association between urinary protein excretion and home BP than office BP. Tanaka et al. [16] conducted a sub-analysis of 228 patients with diabetes who participated in a randomized trial of an angiotensin receptor blocker and a calcium antagonist. They also found a closer association between UACR and home BP than office BP. Matsui et al. examined 356 patients with hypertension that had never been treated [4]. They found that the goodness-of-fit of a model based on mean office SBP with which to predict albuminuria defined as UACR ≥22 and ≥ 31 mg/gCr in men and women, respectively, was significantly improved when mean home SBP was added to the model, as indicated by the likelihood ratio test ($P = 0.006$). Ishikawa et al. examined UACR in 854 patients with cardiovascular risk factors in the Japan Morning Surge-Home Blood Pressure (J-HOP) Study [5]. They reported that the goodness-of-fit of the relationship between systolic BP and UACR was significantly improved by adding home BP measurements taken in the morning and evening to office BP.

3.2.4 Glomerular Filtration Rate (GFR)

One systematic review [3] found that data from four studies [11, 13, 17, 18] were too heterogeneous in terms of populations and methods of GFR estimation to be pooled. To date, the strength of associations between GFR and home and office BP has not been compared.

3.2.5 Pulse Wave Velocity (PWV)

A systematic review [3] found three studies of 720 individuals in which correlation coefficients were investigated between PWV and BP measured at home and in the office [15, 19, 20]. Two and one of the studies measured carotid-femoral [15, 19] and aortic-popliteal PWV [20], respectively. Pooled correlation coefficients did not significantly differ between PWV and home and office BP (0.41 [95% CI: −0.10–0.65]/0.18 [0.17–0.50], $P = 0.18$; vs. 0.35 [0.16–0.52]/0.12 [0.14–0.37], $P = 0.22$). Another recent study also found that adding home BP to a model including office BP did not improve the regression model for carotid-femoral PWV [7].

3.2.6 Silent Cerebrovascular Lesions (SCL)

The Ohasama study by Hara et al. assessed 1007 individuals in a general population [14]. They defined SCL as white matter hyperintensities of grade ≥ 1 or more, lacunar infarcts, or combinations of these findings on MRI images. They reported that the adjusted OR for risk of SCL per 1-SD increase in systolic BP was significantly higher for home than for office BP (22% [95% CI, 4%–42%] vs. 1% [95% CI, −12% to 17%]. No other publications have described an association between home BP and SCL.

3.3 Preclinical Target Organ Damage with Masked Hypertension (MHT) Defined by Home BP

Masked hypertension (MHT) is characterized by BP that is not in the hypertensive range in the office, but is within the hypertensive range when measured out of the office. Although several studies have investigated preclinical target organ damage in patients with MHT, most used ambulatory BP values as out-of-office BP [21]. On the other hand, a few studies that were mostly population-based have shown an association between MHT defined by home BP and preclinical organ damage (Table 3.1).

The Ohasama study examined associations between participants with preclinical carotid atherosclerosis [22], SCL [23], and chronic kidney disease (CKD) [24]. That study found consistently increased risk for preclinical organ damage in participants with MHT compared with participants who had sustained normal BP.

The Finn-Home study examined associations between participants with MHT and preclinical carotid IMT, ECG-LVH, and PWV [25]. That study also found consistently increased risk for preclinical organ damage among participants with MHT compared with participants who had sustained normal BP.

The Hisayama study of associations between preclinical carotid atherosclerosis [26] and CKD [27] found significantly increased risk of carotid atherosclerosis among individuals with MHT compared with participants who sustained normal BP. However, the prevalence of CKD did not significantly differ between participants with MHT and sustained normal BP.

A study of outpatients with CVD risk factors identified significantly higher risk of preclinical organ damage (carotid IMT and brachial-ankle PWV) in those with MHT than with normal BP [28].

Table 3.1 Preclinical target organ damage with masked hypertension (MHT) defined by home BP

Authors	Number of participants	Population characteristics	Methods of home BP measurements	Home BP values analyzed	Preclinical organ damage investigated	Summary of risk associated with MHT
Hara A, et al.	812	General population in Ohasama town, 31% treated	Self-measured once every morning and evening for 4 weeks	Average of 24 morning and 24 evening values	Carotid IMT Carotid plaque	According to morning BP definition, adjusted IMT in individuals with MHT (0.77 mm; 95% CI, 0.73–0.80 mm) was significantly greater than in those with SNBP (0.71 mm; 95% CI, 0.69 to 0.72 mm) ($P < 0.0001$) Significantly higher risk for carotid plaque in MHT compared with SNBP (OR, 1.9; 95% CI, 0.98–3.6) Similar results based on evening home BP
Terawaki H, et al.	1365	General population in Ohasama, 31% treated	Self-measured once every morning for 4 weeks	Average of 26 morning values	CKD (CCr < 60 mL/min with proteinuria)	Significantly higher risk for CKD in MHT (OR, 2.56; 95% CI, 1.11–5.93) than SNBP
Hara A, et al.	1060	General population in Ohasama, 39% treated	Self-measured once every morning and evening for 4 weeks	Average of 49 morning and 49 evening values	SCL	According to morning BP definition, OR of MHT (2.31; 95% CI, 1.32–4.04) for SCL is significantly higher than that for SNBP. Similar results based on evening home BP
Hänninen MR, et al.	1540[a]	Random sample of general population in Finland. Untreated	Self-measured once every morning and evening for 7 days	Average of 27 morning and 27 evening values	Cornell voltage ECG-LVH cIMT PWV	Significantly higher values in MHT compared with SNBP for Cornell voltage (19.0 ± 0.47 vs. 17.2 ± 0.19 mV), ECG-LVH (10.8% vs. 4.4%), cIMT (1.03 ± 0.03 vs. 0.97 ± 0.02 mm) and PWV (14.8 ± 0.61 vs. 13.2 ± 0.51 mm)
Fukuhara M, et al.	2915	General population in Hisayama, 31% treated	Self-measured three times each morning for 4 weeks	Average of 25 morning values	Carotid IMT Carotid stenosis	Geometric average of mean IMT significantly higher among individuals with MHT than normotension (0.77 vs. 0.67 mm; $P < 0.001$). MHT associated with increased likelihood of carotid stenosis compared with normotension (1.95 [1.25–3.03])

(continued)

Table 3.1 (continued)

Authors	Number of participants	Population characteristics	Methods of home BP measurements	Home BP values analyzed	Preclinical organ damage investigated	Summary of risk associated with MHT
Hata J, et al.	2974	General population in Hisayama. 31% treated	Self-measured three times each morning for 4 week	Average of 24 morning values	UACR eGFR CKD (proteinuria and/ or eGFR < 60)	Age- and sex-adjusted geometric mean of UACR values significantly higher in individuals with MHT with SNBP (19.6 vs. 12.5 mg g⁻¹; all $P < 0.001$) MHT significantly associated with increased likelihood of albuminuria compared with NT (26.4% vs. 14.1%; $P < 0.001$) Adjusted mean eGFR did not differ between NT and MHT groups and age- and sex-adjusted mean of eGFR (NT: 70.7 mL/min⁻¹/1.73 m²; 95% CI, 70.0–71.5; MHT: mL/min⁻¹/1.73 m²; 95% CI, 71.1–73.2) Age- and sex-adjusted prevalence of CKD significantly higher in MHT than the NT (36.8% vs. 27.5%). These associations became lost significant after adjustment for other cardiovascular risk factors (multivariable-adjusted OR for MHT vs. NT: 1.20 (0.95–1.52) for MHT vs. NT
Matsui Y, et al.	282	Outpatients in local hospital with CVD risk factors. Untreated	Self-measured three times every morning and evening for 4 days	Average of 24 morning and 24 evening values	Carotid IMT baPWV	IMT was significantly higher in MHT than NT (respective means: 1.01 vs. 0.83 mm, $P < 0.01$). baPWV significantly higher in MHT than NT (mean: 1940 vs. 1733 cm/s, $P < 0.01$)
Tientcheu D	3027	General population in Dallas, 21% treated	Measured 5 times by investigators during daytime home visit	Average of the third to fifth values	APWV Cystatin C UACR	APWV and cystatin C levels significantly higher in MHT than NT (5.39 ± 1.40 vs. 4.56 ± 1.33 m/s and 0.87 ± 0.15 vs. 0.82 ± 0.14 mg/L; $P < 0.01$ for both). Median UACR was also higher in MHT than NT (13 [IQR, 0–34] vs. 2 [IQR, −1 to 15] mg/g creatinine; $P < 0.01$)

CI confidence interval, *CKD* chronic kidney disease, *CVD* cardiovascular disease, *ECG-LVH* electrocardiographic-left ventricular hypertrophy, *eGFR* estimated glomerular filtration rate, *IMT* intima-media thickness, *MHT* masked hypertension, *OR* odds ratio, *SCL* silent cerebrovascular lesion, *SHT* sustained hypertension, *SNBP* sustained normal blood pressure, *PWV* pulse wave velocity, *UACR* urinary albumin-creatinine ratio, *WCHT* white-coat hypertension
[a]IMT and PWV were measured in 592 and 158 participants, respectively

The population-based Dallas heart study found that aortic PWV, UACR, and cystatin C levels were significantly higher in groups with MHT than with normal BP [29]. However, home BP in that study was measured by investigators, not the participants themselves. Therefore, the results should be considered as being quite different from those of other studies in which study participants measured their BP at home.

3.4 Morning vs. Evening Home BP Values with Preclinical Organ Damage

The J-HOP study measured morning and evening HBP, UACR, LVMI, baPWV, maximum carotid IMT, N-terminal pro-brain–type natriuretic peptide (NT-proBNP), and high-sensitivity cardiac troponin T (Hs-cTnT) in 4310 patients with at least one cardiovascular risk factor [30]. They reported that the goodness-of-fit for associations between evening systolic BP and UACR ($P < 0.001$), LVMI ($P < 0.05$), baPWV ($P < 0.001$), NT-proBNP ($P < 0.001$), and Hs-cTnT ($P < 0.001$) was improved by adding morning home systolic BP to systolic BP values, whereas that for associations between morning home systolic BP and UACR ($P < 0.05$) or baPWV ($P < 0.01$) was improved by adding evening home systolic BP to the systolic BP values, indicating that the strength of the association with morning and evening BP differed according to the type of preclinical organ damage.

The Hisayama study examined associations between carotid IMT and BP measured in the morning and evening at home by 2856 community-dwelling individuals aged ≥40 years [31]. They found no differences between them, indicating that both morning and evening home BP were significantly associated with carotid atherosclerosis in that general Japanese population.

Data derived from 464 participants in the Fin-Home study by Johansson et al. found that morning and evening BP were equally closely associated with urinary microalbumin measured by 24-h urine collection [32]. They consequently showed that morning home BP was slightly more closely associated with LVMI than evening home BP.

A study of 561 participants with prehypertension and stage 1 hypertension at 11 medical centers within the Taiwan hypertension-associated cardiac disease consortium [7] measured parameters of target organ damage including LVMI, left atrial volume index (LAVI), and carotid-femoral PWV. The goodness-of-fit of the association between systolic BP and LVMI and LAVI improved by adding morning home systolic BP to the other systolic BP values ($P < 0.001$). They concluded that morning home systolic BP appears to be a better predictor of cardiac damage than any other BP measures in patients with early-stage hypertension.

3.5 Other Topics

Associations between preclinical organ damage and nighttime home BP values and home BP variability are reviewed in Chaps. 13 and 15 of this book, respectively.

3.6   Conclusions

Home BP is closely associated with LVH. However, findings for other types of preclinical target organ damage are inconsistent and/or few studies have been published. Further investigation is needed to compare the strength of associations between other types of preclinical target organ damage, particularly SCL, and home and office BP. In addition, associations between morning and evening BP and preclinical target organ damage also require further investigation.

Associations between MHT determined by self-measured home BP and preclinical target organ damage have been examined only in three population studies and in one study of patients. However, all the findings of these studies revealed a significantly higher prevalent risk of preclinical target organ damage in patients with MHT than in those whose BP was within the normal range. Although the number of studies and the types of preclinical target organ damage investigated were limited, these findings indicate that individuals with advanced preclinical target organ damage and normal office BP values should measure their BP at home for the early detection of MHT.

References

1. Whelton PK, Carey RM, Aronow WS, Casey DE Jr, Collins KJ, Dennison Himmelfarb C, et al. 2017 ACC/AHA/AAPA/ABC/ACPM/AGS/APhA/ASH/ASPC/NMA/PCNA Guideline for the Prevention, Detection, Evaluation, and Management of High Blood Pressure in Adults: a report of the American College of Cardiology/American Heart Association Task Force on Clinical Practice Guidelines. Hypertension. 2018;71(6):e13–e115.
2. Williams B, Mancia G, Spiering W, Agabiti Rosei E, Azizi M, Burnier M, et al. 2018 ESC/ESH guidelines for the management of arterial hypertension: the task force for the management of arterial hypertension of the European Society of Cardiology and the European Society of Hypertension. J Hypertens. 2018;36(10):1953–2041.
3. Bliziotis I, Destounis A, Stergiou GS. Home versus ambulatory and office blood pressure in predicting target organ damage in hypertension: a systematic review and meta-analysis. J Hypertens. 2012;30(7):1289–99.
4. Matsui Y, Ishikawa J, Eguchi K, Shibasaki S, Shimada K, Kario K. Maximum value of home blood pressure: a novel indicator of target organ damage in hypertension. Hypertension. 2011;57(6):1087–93.
5. Ishikawa J, Hoshide S, Eguchi K, Ishikawa S, Shimada K, Kario K. Japan morning surge-home blood pressure study investigators group. Nighttime home blood pressure and the risk of hypertensive target organ damage. Hypertension. 2012;60(4):921–8.
6. Her AY, Kim YH, Rim SJ, Kim JY, Choi EY, Min PK, Lee BK, Hong BK, Kwon HM. Home blood pressure is the predictor of subclinical target organ damage like ambulatory blood pressure monitoring in untreated hypertensive patients. Anadolu Kardiyol Derg. 2014;14(8):711–8.
7. Lin TT, Juang JJ, Lee JK, Tsai CT, Chen CH, Yu WC, et al. Comparison of home and ambulatory blood pressure measurements in association with preclinical hypertensive cardiovascular damage. J Cardiovasc Nurs. 2019;34(2):106–14.
8. Siven SS, Niiranen TJ, Langen VL, Puukka PJ, Kantola IM, Jula AM. Home versus office blood pressure: longitudinal relations with left ventricular hypertrophy: the Finn-Home study. J Hypertens. 2017;35(2):266–71.

9. Mancia G, Zanchetti A, Agabiti-Rosei E, Benemio G, De Cesaris R, Fogari R, et al. Ambulatory blood pressure is superior to clinic blood pressure in predicting treatment-induced regression of left ventricular hypertrophy. SAMPLE study group. Study on ambulatory monitoring of blood pressure and Lisinopril evaluation. Circulation. 1997;95(6):1464–70.

10. Martínez MA, Sancho T, García P, Moreno P, Rubio JM, Palau FJ, et al. Home blood pressure in poorly controlled hypertension: relationship with ambulatory blood pressure and organ damage. Blood Press Monit. 2006;11(4):207–13.

11. Gaborieau V, Delarche N, Gosse P. Ambulatory blood pressure monitoring versus self-measurement of blood pressure at home: correlation with target organ damage. J Hypertens. 2008;26(10):1919–27.

12. Tachibana R, Tabara Y, Kondo I, Miki T, Kohara K. Home blood pressure is a better predictor of carotid atherosclerosis than office blood pressure in community-dwelling subjects. Hypertens Res. 2004;27(9):633–9.

13. Niiranen T, Jula A, Kantola I, Moilanen L, Kähönen M, Kesäniemi YA, et al. Home-measured blood pressure is more strongly associated with atherosclerosis than clinic blood pressure: the Finn-HOME study. J Hypertens. 2007;25(6):1225–31.

14. Hara A, Tanaka K, Ohkubo T, Kondo T, Kikuya M, Metoki H, et al. Ambulatory versus home versus clinic blood pressure: the association with subclinical cerebrovascular diseases: the Ohasama study. Hypertension. 2012;59(1):22–8.

15. Stergiou GS, Argyraki KK, Moyssakis I, Mastorantonakis SE, Achimastos AD, Karamanos VG, et al. Home blood pressure is as reliable as ambulatory blood pressure in predicting target-organ damage in hypertension. Am J Hypertens. 2007;20(6):616–21.

16. Tanaka Y, Daida H, Imai Y, Miyauchi K, Sato Y, Hiwatari M, et al. Morning home blood pressure may be a significant marker of nephropathy in Japanese patients with type 2 diabetes: ADVANCED-J study 1. Hypertens Res. 2009;32(9):770–4.

17. Kuriyama S, Otsuka Y, Iida R, Matsumoto K, Tokudome G, Hosoya T. Morning blood pressure predicts hypertensive organ damage in patients with renal diseases: effect of intensive antihypertensive therapy in patients with diabetic nephropathy. Intern Med. 2005;44(12):1239–46.

18. Okada T, Nakao T, Matsumoto H, Nagaoka Y, Tomaru R, Iwasawa H, et al. Prognostic significance of home blood pressure control on renal and cardiovascular outcomes in elderly patients with chronic kidney disease. Hypertens Res. 2009;32(12):1123–9.

19. Calvo-Vargas C, Padilla-Rios V, Meza-Flores A, Vazquez-Linares G, Troyo-Sanromán R, Cerda AP, et al. Arterial stiffness and blood pressure self-measurement with loaned equipment. Am J Hypertens. 2003;16(5 Pt 1):375–80.

20. Niiranen TJ, Jula AM, Kantola IM, Kähönen M, Reunanen A. Home blood pressure has a stronger association with arterial stiffness than clinic blood pressure: the Finn-Home Study. Blood Press Monit. 2009;14(5):196–201.

21. Cuspidi C, Sala C, Tadic M, Rescaldani M, Grassi G, Mancia G. Untreated masked hypertension and subclinical cardiac damage: a systematic review and meta-analysis. Am J Hypertens. 2015;28(6):806–13.

22. Hara A, Ohkubo T, Kikuya M, Shintani Y, Obara T, Metoki H, et al. Detection of carotid atherosclerosis in individuals with masked hypertension and white-coat hypertension by self-measured blood pressure at home: the Ohasama study. J Hypertens. 2007;25(2):321–7.

23. Hara A, Ohkubo T, Kondo T, Kikuya M, Aono Y, Hanawa S, et al. Detection of silent cerebrovascular lesions in individuals with 'masked' and 'white-coat' hypertension by home blood pressure measurement: the Ohasama study. J Hypertens. 2009;27(5):1049–55.

24. Terawaki H, Metoki H, Nakayama M, Ohkubo T, Kikuya M, Asayama K, et al. Masked hypertension determined by self-measured blood pressure at home and chronic kidney disease in the Japanese general population: the Ohasama study. Hypertens Res. 2008;31(12):2129–35.

25. Hanninen MR, Niiranen TJ, Puukka PJ, Kesaniemi YA, Kahonen M, Jula AM. Target organ damage and masked hypertension in the general population: the Finn-home study. J Hypertens. 2013;31(6):1136–43.

26. Fukuhara M, Arima H, Ninomiya T, Hata J, Hirakawa Y, Doi Y, et al. White-coat and masked hypertension are associated with carotid atherosclerosis in a general population: the Hisayama study. Stroke. 2013;44(6):1512–7.
27. Hata J, Fukuhara M, Sakata S, Arima H, Hirakawa Y, Yonemoto K, et al. White-coat and masked hypertension are associated with albuminuria in a general population: the Hisayama study. Hypertens Res. 2017;40(11):937–43.
28. Matsui Y, Eguchi K, Ishikawa J, Hoshide S, Shimada K, Kario K. Subclinical arterial damage in untreated masked hypertensive subjects detected by home blood pressure measurement. Am J Hypertens. 2007;20(4):385–91.
29. Tientcheu D, Ayers C, Das SR, McGuire DK, de Lemos JA, Khera A, et al. Target organ complications and cardiovascular events associated with masked hypertension and white-coat hypertension: analysis from the Dallas Heart Study. J Am Coll Cardiol. 2015;66(20):2159–69.
30. Hoshide S, Kario K, Yano Y, Haimoto H, Yamagiwa K, Uchiba K, et al. Association of morning and evening blood pressure at home with asymptomatic organ damage in the J-HOP study. Am J Hypertens. 2014;27(7):939–47.
31. Sakata S, Hata J, Fukuhara M, Yonemoto K, Mukai N, Yoshida D, et al. Morning and evening blood pressures are associated with intima-media thickness in a general population- the Hisayama study. Circ J. 2017;81(11):1647–53.
32. Johansson JK, Niiranen TJ, Puukka PJ, Jula AM. Optimal schedule for home blood pressure monitoring based on a clinical approach. J Hypertens. 2010;28(2):259–64.

Home Blood Pressure as Predictor of Adverse Health Outcomes

4

Kei Asayama, Teemu J. Niiranen, Takayoshi Ohkubo, George S. Stergiou, Lutgarde Thijs, Yutaka Imai, and Jan A. Staessen

K. Asayama (✉)
Department of Hygiene and Public Health, Teikyo University School of Medicine, Tokyo, Japan

Tohoku Institute for Management of Blood Pressure, Sendai, Japan

Studies Coordinating Centre, Research Unit Hypertension and Cardiovascular Epidemiology, KU Leuven Department of Cardiovascular Sciences, University of Leuven, Leuven, Belgium
e-mail: kei@asayama.org

T. J. Niiranen
Department of Public Health Solutions, National Institute for Health and Welfare, Turku, Finland

Department of Medicine, Turku University Hospital and University of Turku, Turku, Finland
e-mail: teemu.niiranen@thl.fi

T. Ohkubo
Department of Hygiene and Public Health, Teikyo University School of Medicine, Tokyo, Japan

Tohoku Institute for Management of Blood Pressure, Sendai, Japan
e-mail: tohkubo@med.teikyo-u.ac.jp

G. S. Stergiou
Hypertension Center STRIDE-7, National and Kapodistrian University of Athens, School of Medicine, Third Department of Medicine, Sotiria Hospital, Athens, Greece
e-mail: gstergi@med.uoa.gr

L. Thijs
Studies Coordinating Centre, Research Unit Hypertension and Cardiovascular Epidemiology, KU Leuven Department of Cardiovascular Sciences, University of Leuven, Leuven, Belgium
e-mail: lutgarde.thijs@kuleuven.be

Y. Imai
Tohoku Institute for Management of Blood Pressure, Sendai, Japan
e-mail: yutaka.imai.d6@tohoku.ac.jp

J. A. Staessen
Studies Coordinating Centre, Research Unit Hypertension and Cardiovascular Epidemiology, KU Leuven Department of Cardiovascular Sciences, University of Leuven, Leuven, Belgium

Cardiovascular Research Institute Maastricht (CARIM), Maastricht University, Maastricht, The Netherlands
e-mail: jan.staessen@kuleuven.be

© The Editor(s), under exclusive license to Springer Nature Switzerland AG 2020
G. S. Stergiou et al. (eds.), *Home Blood Pressure Monitoring*,
Updates in Hypertension and Cardiovascular Protection,
https://doi.org/10.1007/978-3-030-23065-4_4

4.1   Introduction

In the 1970s, home blood pressure measurement made its entry in clinical research [1, 2]. In the late 1980s, automated cuff-oscillometric home blood pressure monitors entered the market. Subsequently, studies highlighting the prognostic accuracy of the self-measured home blood pressure in populations and patients have paved the way for the widespread clinical application of this approach. The Lancet Commission on hypertension proposed better assessment of blood pressure as one of the key measures to be implemented to stop what has been named *the largest epidemic ever known to mankind* [3]. In this chapter, we review the prognostic studies regarding self-measured home blood pressure (Table 4.1), and clarify that self-measurement of the blood pressure at home is required to achieve the goal [3]. For the sake of comparability, we converted reported hazard ratios to express relative risk associated with a 10/5-mm Hg increment in systolic/diastolic blood pressure, when blood pressure was analysed on a continuous scale.

4.2   General Population

The Ohasama study (Hanamaki, Japan), initiated in 1986, is the first population study focusing on the prognostic accuracy of the self-measured home blood pressure. As reported in 1998, in Cox proportional hazard models including both the conventional office blood pressure and home blood pressure, the mean of multiple home systolic pressure measurements predicted cardiovascular mortality over and beyond the conventional systolic pressure (hazard ratio, 1.22; 95% confidence interval [CI], 1.00–1.48) [4]. While in the Ohasama cohort the incidence of stroke was closer associated with a single morning or evening home blood pressure on the first

Table 4.1 Characteristics of studies investigating cardiovascular outcome based on self-measured home blood pressure

Study type	Study name	Publication Year (ref)	Country	Sample size	Follow-up (years)
General population	Ohasama	1998 [4]	Japan	1789	6.6
	PAMELA	2005[14]	Italy	2051	10.9
	Didima	2007[11]	Greece	662	8.2
	Finn-Home	2010[13]	Finland	2081	6.8
Patient study	SHEAF	2004 [15]	France	4939	3.0
	HOMED-BP	2012 [16]	Japan	3518	5.3
	HONEST	2014 [18]	Japan	21,591	2.0
	J-HOP	2016 [19]	Japan	4278	4.0
Meta-Analysis	IDHOCO	2013 [21]	Multiple	6470	8.3

Publication year represents the first peer-reviewed publication. *PAMELA* the Pressioni Arteriose Monitorate e Loro Associazioni, *SHEAF* Self-Measurement of Blood Pressure at Home in the Elderly: Assessment and Follow-up, *HOMED-BP* Hypertension Objective Treatment Based on Measurement by Electrical Devices of Blood Pressures, *HONEST* Olmesartan Naive patients to Establish Standard Target blood pressure, *J-HOP* the Japan Morning Surge-Home Blood Pressure, *IDHOCO* the International Database of HOme blood pressure in relation to Cardiovascular Outcome

monitoring day than the conventional blood pressure, the predictive accuracy of the home blood pressure increased with the number of monitoring days up to 2 weeks [5, 6]. The Ohasama investigators also reported the incidence of stroke according to the level of the office and home blood pressures after stratification for cardiovascular risk based on the criteria proposed by contemporary European and American guidelines [7, 8]. The key points emerging from these analyses (Fig. 4.1) were that

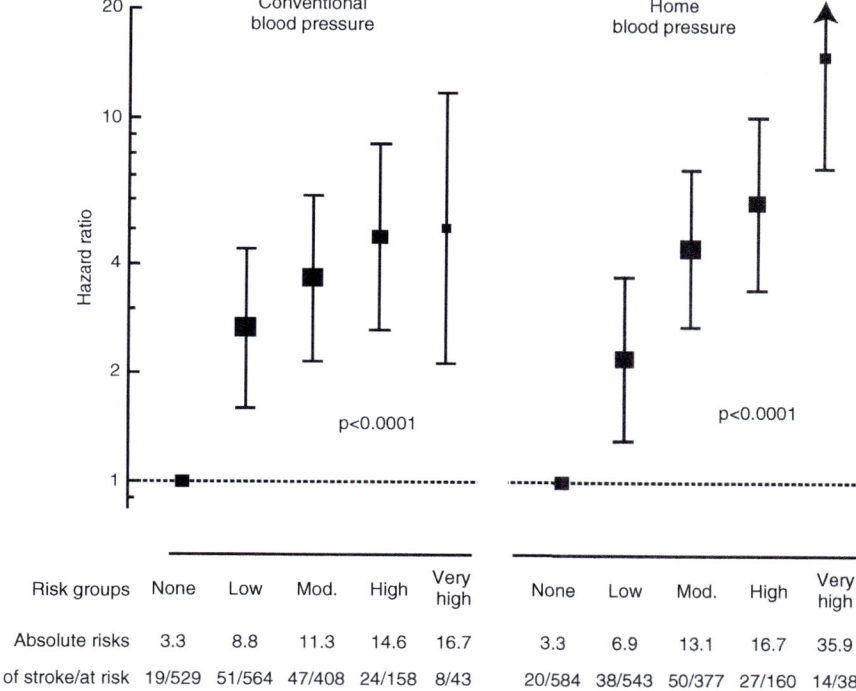

Risk groups	None	Low	Mod.	High	Very high	None	Low	Mod.	High	Very high
Absolute risks	3.3	8.8	11.3	14.6	16.7	3.3	6.9	13.1	16.7	35.9
N° of stroke/at risk	19/529	51/564	47/408	24/158	8/43	20/584	38/543	50/377	27/160	14/38

Fig. 4.1 Risk of stroke according to the multiple risk factor classification proposed by the 2003 European hypertension guideline. Risk factors include either the conventional or the self-measured blood pressure at home. The participants were first classified into one of six blood pressure categories as optimal (home, 115/75 mmHg; conventional, 120/80 mmHg), normal (home, 115/75–124/79 mmHg; conventional, 120/80–129/84 mmHg), high normal (home, 125/80–134/84 mmHg; conventional, 130/85–139/89 mmHg), grade 1 (home, 135/85–149/94 mmHg; conventional, 140/90–159/99 mmHg), grade 2 (home, 150/95–164/104 mmHg; conventional, 160/100–179/109 mmHg), or grade 3 hypertension (home, ≥165/105; conventional, ≥180/110 mmHg) based on the rate of participants from each level of home and conventional blood pressure classification. Based on the combination of the six blood pressure categories and the extent of cardiovascular risks—no risk factors, one or two risk factors, ≥2 risk factors or diabetes mellitus, or past history of cardiovascular disease—, they were finally assigned to one of five risk groups according to the 2003 European guidelines criteria, from none (reference group) to very high risk groups. Participants classified according to conventional and home blood pressure were analysed separately. The absolute risk is expressed in stroke events per 1000 person-years. Squares and vertical lines indicate the point estimate and 95% confidence interval of the hazard ratio in each subgroup, the size of the square being proportional to the number of events. p values are for trend across risk subgroups. Reproduced with permission from Asayama et al. [7]

even in patients with low added risk both the office and self-measured blood pressures predicted stroke, and that across the strata of cardiovascular risk the probability of a first stroke rose steeper with the home than with the conventional blood pressure [7]. Among treated patients with hypertension enrolled in the Ohasama population study, the risk of stroke remained associated with the home blood pressure, but not with the conventional blood pressure [9]. Another analysis of Ohasama data demonstrated that morning and evening blood pressure were equally predictive of stroke in all participants, but that morning compared with evening blood pressure was a better predictor in treated than untreated hypertensive patients, perhaps as a consequence of the dosing of antihypertensive drugs in the morning after measurement of the morning blood pressure [10].

The Didima study (Greece), initiated in 1997, involved 662 of its residents (58.2% women; mean age at enrolment, 54.1 years) [11]. Over 8.2 years of follow-up, 78 deaths, 42 of cardiovascular causes, and 67 fatal and non-fatal cardiovascular events occurred. The unadjusted hazard ratios for cardiovascular events were 1.41 ($p < 0.001$) and 1.40 ($p < 0.001$) for conventional office systolic and home systolic pressure, respectively; the corresponding estimates for diastolic pressure were 1.20 ($p < 0.01$) and 1.11 ($p = 0.07$). In contrast to the Ohasama findings [4], addition of the home blood pressure (average of duplicate readings in the morning and evening on three consecutive days) to Cox models already including the office blood pressure (average of six readings; three readings at each of two clinic visits) did not significantly improve the prediction of cardiovascular complications [11]. Confirmatory findings when the Didima participants were further followed-up for totalled 19.0 years, with 216 deaths (127 cardiovascular causes) and 174 cardiovascular events occurred, were later reported [12].

The Finn-Home study included 2081 individuals aged 45 to 74 years, representative for the whole of Finland [13]. After 6.8 years of follow-up, 162 participants had experienced a cardiovascular event. In multivariable-adjusted analyses, the systolic/diastolic hazard ratios were 1.13/1.13 (CI, 1.05–1.22/1.05–1.22) for conventional office blood pressure and 1.23/1.18 (CI, 1.13–1.34/1.10–1.27) for home blood pressure. However, when both types of blood pressure estimates were simultaneously entered in the models, only the hazard ratios for home blood pressure (1.22/1.15; 1.09–1.37/1.05–1.26), not office blood pressure (1.01/1.06; CI, 0.92–1.12/0.97–1.16), retained significance.

High prognostic ability of 1-day home blood pressure measurements for cardiovascular mortality was reported from the Pressioni Arteriose Monitorate e Loro Associazioni (PAMELA) study [14]. Among 2051 Italian participants, 56 of 186 observed deaths during 11.9 years of follow-up were cardiovascular. Risk of cardiovascular death increased more with a given increase in home than in conventional blood pressure, and a significant improvement of the prediction model was obtained by adding home blood pressure to the initial model with conventional blood pressure (Goodness of Fit, 15.039; $p < 0.001$) [14].

4.3   Patient Studies

The "Self-Measurement of Blood Pressure at Home in the Elderly: Assessment and Follow-up" (SHEAF) study involved a 3-year follow-up of 4939 patients with anti-hypertensive drug treatment in general practice (women, 51.1%; mean age, 70.0 years), who experienced 324 cardiovascular endpoints [15]. The systolic/dia-stolic multivariable-adjusted hazard ratios for home blood pressure were 1.17/1.12 (CI, 1.11–1.24/1.06–1.18), whereas the corresponding associations with the office blood pressure were not significant ($p \geq 0.09$). In a multivariable model with patients having controlled hypertension as the reference, the hazard ratios were 2.06 (CI, 1.22–3.47) in patients with normal office blood pressure (threshold 140/90 mmHg) and elevated home blood pressure (threshold 135/85 mm Hg), 1.18 (CI, 0.67–2.10) in patients with elevated office, but normal home blood pressure, and 1.96 (CI, 1.27–3.02) in patients with elevated blood pressure on both types of measurement.

The multicentre Hypertension Objective Treatment Based on Measurement by Electrical Devices of Blood Pressure (HOMED-BP) included 3518 patients (women, 50%; mean age, 59.6 years) [16]. Over 5.3 years of follow-up, the major adverse cardiovascular event consisting of cardiovascular death, stroke and myocardial infarction occurred in 51 participants. In fully adjusted models, the hazard ratios associated with systolic home blood pressure before the initiation of antihyperten-sive drug treatment and on treatment were 1.32 (CI, 1.05–1.66) and 1.34 (CI, 1.11–1.61), respectively [16]. There was a log-linear increase of the risk across thirds of the distributions of the untreated home systolic pressure at baseline and the achieved home systolic pressure during follow-up (Fig. 4.2) [17]. Across thirds of the base-line systolic pressure before treatment, levels averaged 138.2, 150.4 and 166.1 mmHg; the corresponding mean levels on treatment were 116.8, 128.2 and 144.4 mmHg. These observations highlight the potential of monitoring blood pres-sure at home before and after initiation of antihypertensive drug treatment as well as the importance of strict blood pressure control.

The Olmesartan Naive patients to Establish Standard Target blood pressure (HONEST) study [18] was a surveillance of 21,591 patients (women, 50.6%; mean age, 64.9 years) receiving the angiotensin receptor blocker olmesartan on top of other antihypertensive drugs. After 2 years of follow-up, 280 cardiovascular events had occurred. Patients with morning home systolic blood pressure 145 mmHg or higher had a significantly higher risk (hazard ratio, 2.47; CI, 1.20–5.08) than patients with morning home systolic blood pressure of less than 125 mmHg. The Japan Morning Surge-Home Blood Pressure (J-HOP) study confirmed the prognostic accuracy of the morning blood pressure [19]. This multicentre study involved 4278 patients with a history of and/or risk factors for cardiovascular disease (women, 65.6%; mean age 64.9 years). Over a mean follow-up of 4.0 years, stroke or coro-nary artery disease had occurred in 74 and 77 patients, respectively. The morning systolic pressure improved the discrimination of incident stroke (C statistics, 0.802; CI, 0.692–0.911) beyond traditional risk factors, including office systolic pressure (C statistics, 0.756; CI, 0.646–0.866); this was not the case for prediction of coro-nary artery disease. In the same J-HOP population [19], masked hypertension

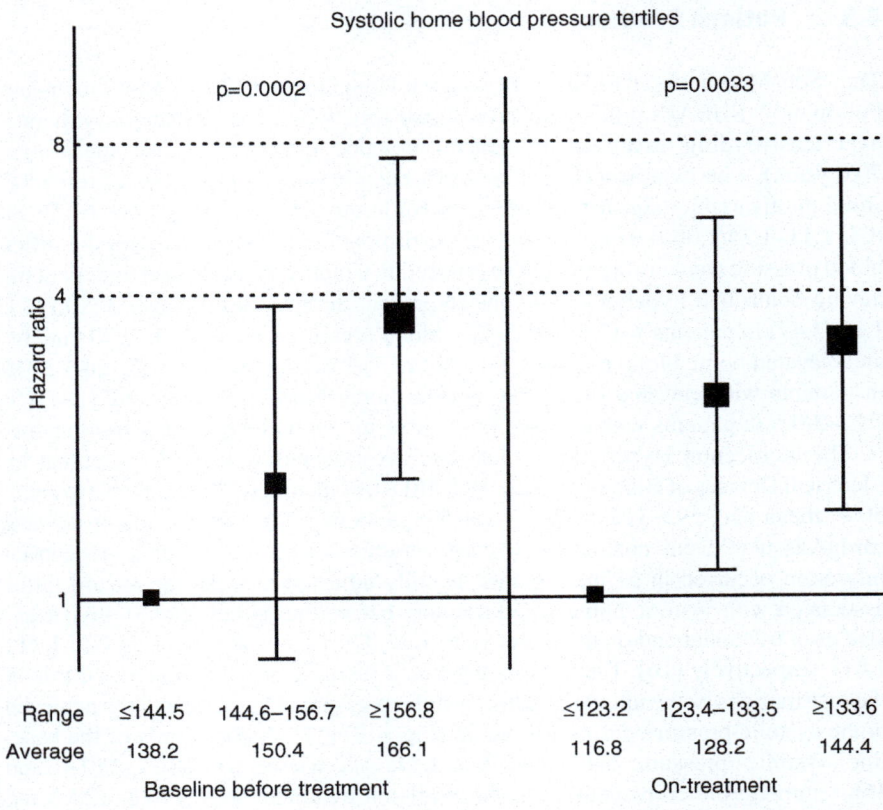

Fig. 4.2 Hazard ratios for major adverse cardiovascular events across thirds of the pretreatment (left) and on-treatment (right) home systolic pressure. Squares representing the hazard ratios are sized proportionally to the number of cardiovascular endpoints. Vertical bars indicate 95% confidence intervals for comparison with the lowest third. For each plotted point, the range and average of the home systolic pressure are given (mm Hg). p values express the significance of the log-linear trend. The analyses accounted for sex, age, body mass index, hypercholesterolaemia, smoking and drinking, diabetes mellitus and history of cardiovascular disease. Models including the pretreatment blood pressure were adjusted for the on-treatment blood pressure and vice versa. Reproduced with permission from Asayama et al. [17]

diagnosed based on the 14-day averaged morning and evening home blood pressures was associated with higher stroke risk (hazard ratio for masked hypertension vs. normotension on office and home measurement, 2.77; CI, 1.20–6.37) [20].

4.4 The IDHOCO Participant-Level Meta-Analysis

The International Database of HOme blood pressure in relation to Cardiovascular Outcome (IDHOCO) is a collaborating research project involving seven population studies (in 2018) where participants had measured their home blood pressure and follow-up data with fatal and non-fatal outcomes were fully supplied [21]. Based on the 6470 participants (women, 56.9%; mean age, 59.3 years), we determined home blood pressure thresholds, which yielded 10-year cardiovascular risks similar to those associated with stages 1 (120/80 mmHg) and 2 (130/85 mmHg) prehypertension, and stages 1 (140/90 mmHg) and 2 (160/100 mmHg) hypertension on conventional office measurement [21]. During a median of 8.3 years of follow-up, 716 cardiovascular endpoints occurred. The rounded outcome-driven systolic/diastolic thresholds for the home blood pressure corresponding with stages 1 and 2 prehypertension and stages 1 and 2 hypertension amounted to 120/75, 125/80, 130/85, and 145/90 mmHg, respectively. Population-based outcome-driven thresholds for home blood pressure are slightly lower than those provided in contemporary hypertension guidelines [22, 23].

The continuous nature of the relation with blood pressure not only holds true in hypertensive patients, but in normotensive people as well. Among 5008 untreated participants in the IDHOCO database (women, 56.6%; mean age, 57.1 years) [24], using 135/85 mm Hg as a threshold for the home blood pressure, the number with masked hypertension amounted to 42 (3.1%), 131 (12.9%), and 233 (22.5%) among participants with optimal (<120/<80 mmHg), normal (120–129/80–80 mmHg), and high-normal (130–139/85–89 mmHg) conventional blood pressure. Across these three categories of patients with masked hypertension (Fig. 4.3), using optimal conventional blood pressure without masked hypertension as reference, the

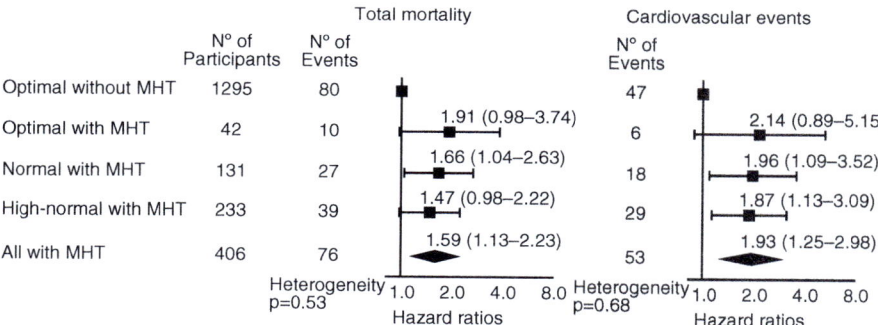

Fig. 4.3 Hazard ratios associated with masked hypertension (MHT; ≥135/85 mm Hg) on home blood pressure monitoring in participants with optimal, normal, or high-normal office blood pressure. Participants with optimal blood pressure without elevated home blood pressure was the reference group. Systolic/diastolic thresholds for the conventional blood pressure were optimal (<120/80 mm Hg), normal (120–129/80–84 mm Hg), and high-normal (130–139/85–89 mm Hg). When a systolic or diastolic blood pressure was in a different category, the participant was assigned to the higher category. Systolic/diastolic thresholds for hypertension on home measurement were ≥ 135/85 mm Hg. The hazard ratios were adjusted for cohort, sex, age, body mass index, smoking, total cholesterol, diabetes mellitus, and history of cardiovascular disease. Horizontal lines denote the 95% confidence interval. The diamond represents the pooled estimate in all patients with MHT. The p value for heterogeneity was derived by testing an ordinal variable in Cox proportional hazard regression coding for the 3 subgroups among patients with MHT. Reproduced with permission from Asayama et al. [24]

multivariable-adjusted hazard ratios for a composite cardiovascular endpoint were 2.14 (CI, 0.89–5.15), 1.96 (CI, 1.09–3.52), and 1.87 (CI, 1.13–3.09), respectively. Thus, home blood pressure refines risk stratification in apparently healthy people with a normal or high-normal office blood pressure, and is therefore an essential information to diagnose hypertension and to initiate or adjust antihypertensive drug treatment.

The IDHOCO database of diverse populations enables us to provide robust subgroup analysis beyond each cohort. Multivariable-adjusted analysis with a bootstrap procedure to determine home blood pressure levels yielding 10-year cardiovascular risks similar to those associated with established systolic/diastolic thresholds for the conventional blood pressure supported that single blood pressure thresholds can be indiscriminately applied in both sexes and across the age range up to 80 years of age [25]. A systolic home blood pressure of 152 mmHg or more and a diastolic home blood pressure of less than 65 mmHg entailed increased cardiovascular risk, whereas a diastolic home blood pressure above 82 mmHg minimized risk among untreated octogenarians [26]. In treated octogenarians in which overtreatment is certainly an issue, total mortality was curvilinearly associated with systolic home blood pressure, i.e., levels below 127 mmHg were associated with increased total mortality with 149 mmHg being associated with lowest risk of death.

4.5   Variability in the Home Blood Pressure

The HOMED-BP extended dataset (median of 7.4 years follow-up) allowed studying the association between a composite cardiovascular endpoint and seasonal variability in the home blood pressure [27]. The study investigators defined seasonal variability as an average of all increases in home blood pressure from summer to winter combined with all decreases in home blood pressure from winter to summer throughout the follow-up period. Compared with the small-to-middle seasonal variability in the home blood pressure (0–9.1/0–4.5 mm Hg), composite cardiovascular outcome was worse in the large variability group (≥9.1/≥4.5 mm Hg; hazard ratio, 2.02/1.95; CI, 1.03–3.97/1.00–3.79) as well as in the inverse variability group (<0/<0 mm Hg; hazard ratio, 3.07/2.81; CI, 1.44–6.54/1.41–5.61) variability group (Fig. 4.4) [27].

Day-to-day (day-by-day) home blood pressure variability in relation to cardiovascular complications is described in Chap. 15 "Home BP Variability". Meanwhile, the day-to-day home blood pressure variability is considered to be a risk factor for the development of cognitive decline [28] and dementia [29]. After a median 7.8 years of follow-up of the 485 Ohasama participants (women, 71.8%; mean age, 63.3 years), home systolic pressure at baseline was significantly associated with cognitive decline ($n = 46$; odds ratio, 1.31; CI, 1.03–1.65) [28]. However, the conventional systolic pressure was not (odds ratio, 1.12; CI, 0.95–1.32) [28]. Furthermore, cognitive decline was positively associated with the day-to-day standard deviation of home systolic pressure in models including the home systolic

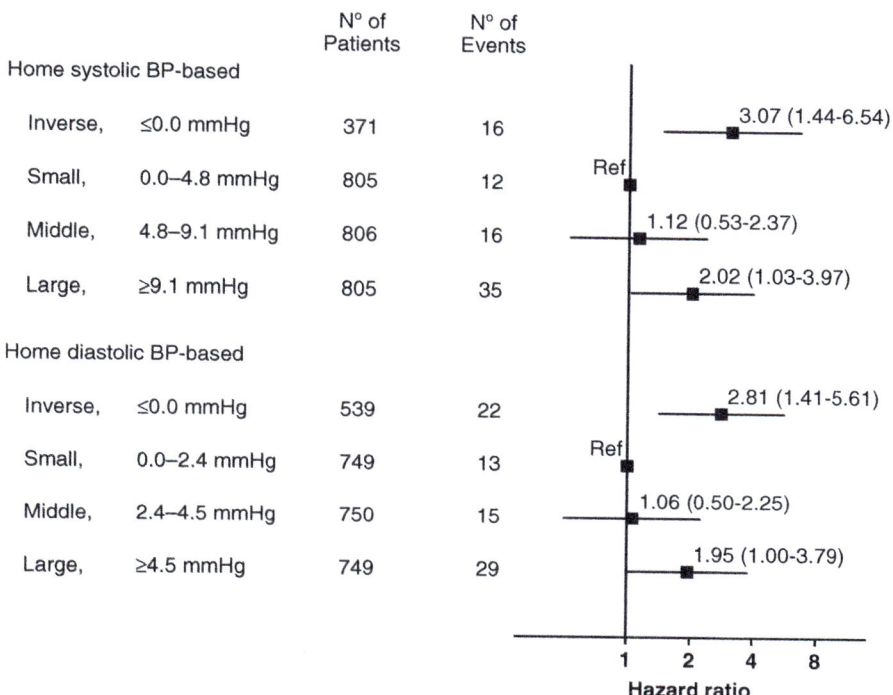

		N° of Patients	N° of Events
Home systolic BP-based			
Inverse,	≤0.0 mmHg	371	16
Small,	0.0–4.8 mmHg	805	12
Middle,	4.8–9.1 mmHg	806	16
Large,	≥9.1 mmHg	805	35
Home diastolic BP-based			
Inverse,	≤0.0 mmHg	539	22
Small,	0.0–2.4 mmHg	749	13
Middle,	2.4–4.5 mmHg	750	15
Large,	≥4.5 mmHg	749	29

Hazard ratios (with 95% CI):
- Home systolic, Inverse: 3.07 (1.44–6.54)
- Home systolic, Small: Ref
- Home systolic, Middle: 1.12 (0.53–2.37)
- Home systolic, Large: 2.02 (1.03–3.97)
- Home diastolic, Inverse: 2.81 (1.41–5.61)
- Home diastolic, Small: Ref
- Home diastolic, Middle: 1.06 (0.50–2.25)
- Home diastolic, Large: 1.95 (1.00–3.79)

Hazard ratio axis: 1 2 4 8

Fig. 4.4 Hazard ratios associated with seasonal home blood pressure (BP) variability for a composite cardiovascular outcome.The seasonal variability in an individual was defined as an average of observed seasonal changes in home blood pressure, i.e., all increases in home blood pressure from summer (July–August) to winter (January–February) combined with all decreases from winter to summer throughout the follow-up period. Hazard ratios for comparison with the reference group were given with 95% confidence interval with adjustments applied for sex, age, the pretreatment and on-treatment home blood pressure, body mass index, smoking and drinking, hypercholesterolaemia, diabetes mellitus and history of cardiovascular disease. Reproduced with permission from Hanazawa et al. [27]

pressure level (odds ratio per 2.6 mmHg increase of SD, 1.51; CI, 1.07–2.12) [28]. The Hisayama study involved a population-based cohort recruited in Fukuoka, Japan [29]. Over a follow-up of 5.3 years, 194 of 1674 participants all aged 60 years or more (women, 55.9%) developed vascular or neurodegenerative dementia. Compared with participants in the bottom fourth of the distribution of the coefficient of variation, the risks of dementia was significantly higher in those in top fourth (multivariable-adjusted hazard ratio, 2.27; CI, 1.45–3.55), thereby confirming the Ohasama results [28].

Acknowledgments We gratefully acknowledge the clerical staff Sachiko Matsuda and Misa Kimura of the Department of Hygiene and Public Health, Teikyo University School of Medicine for their valuable support.

References

1. Staessen JA, Li Y, Hara A, Asayama K, Dolan E, O'Brien E. Blood pressure measurement anno 2016. Am J Hypertens. 2017;30:453–63.
2. Staessen JA, Thijs L, Ohkubo T, Kikuya M, Richart T, Boggia J, et al. Thirty years of research on diagnostic and therapeutic thresholds for the self-measured blood pressure at home. Blood Press Monit. 2008;13:352–65.
3. Yusuf S, Wood D, Ralston J, Reddy KS. The World Heart Federation's vision for worldwide cardiovascular disease prevention. Lancet. 2015;386:399–402.
4. Ohkubo T, Imai Y, Tsuji I, Nagai K, Kato J, Kikuchi N, et al. Home blood pressure measurement has a stronger predictive power for mortality than does screening blood pressure measurement: a population-based observation in Ohasama, Japan. J Hypertens. 1998;16:971–5.
5. Ohkubo T, Asayama K, Kikuya M, Metoki H, Hoshi H, Hashimoto J, et al. How many times should blood pressure be measured at home for better prediction of stroke risk? Ten-year follow-up results from the Ohasama study. J Hypertens. 2004;22:1099–104.
6. Asayama K, Ohkubo T, Hara A, Hirose T, Yasui D, Obara T, et al. Repeated evening home blood pressure measurement improves prognostic significance for stroke: a 12-year follow-up of the Ohasama study. Blood Press Monit. 2009;14:93–8.
7. Asayama K, Ohkubo T, Kikuya M, Metoki H, Obara T, Hoshi H, et al. Use of 2003 European Society of Hypertension-European Society of Cardiology guidelines for predicting stroke using self-measured blood pressure at home: the Ohasama study. Eur Heart J. 2005;26:2026–31.
8. Asayama K, Ohkubo T, Kikuya M, Metoki H, Hoshi H, Hashimoto J, et al. Prediction of stroke by self-measurement of blood pressure at home versus casual screening blood pressure measurement in relation to the JNC-7 classification: the Ohasama study. Stroke. 2004;35:2356–61.
9. Yasui D, Asayama K, Ohkubo T, Kikuya M, Kanno A, Hara A, et al. Stroke risk in treated hypertension based on home blood pressure: the Ohasama study. Am J Hypertens. 2010;23:508–14.
10. Asayama K, Ohkubo T, Kikuya M, Obara T, Metoki H, Inoue R, et al. Prediction of stroke by home "morning" versus "evening" blood pressure values: the Ohasama study. Hypertension. 2006;48:737–43.
11. Stergiou GS, Baibas NM, Kalogeropoulos PG. Cardiovascular risk prediction based on home blood pressure measurement: the Didima study. J Hypertens. 2007;25:1590–6.
12. Ntineri A, Kalogeropoulos PG, Kyriakoulis KG, Aissopou EK, Thomopoulou G, Kollias A, et al. Prognostic value of average home blood pressure and variability: 19-year follow-up of the Didima study. J Hypertens. 2018;36:69–76.
13. Niiranen TJ, Hanninen MR, Johansson J, Reunanen A, Jula AM. Home-measured blood pressure is a stronger predictor of cardiovascular risk than office blood pressure: the Finn-Home study. Hypertension. 2010;55:1346–51.
14. Sega R, Facchetti R, Bombelli M, Cesana G, Corrao G, Grassi G, et al. Prognostic value of ambulatory and home blood pressures compared with office blood pressure in the general population: follow-up results from the Pressioni Arteriose Monitorate e Loro Associazioni (PAMELA) study. Circulation. 2005;111:1777–83.
15. Bobrie G, Chatellier G, Genes N, Clerson P, Vaur L, Vaisse B, et al. Cardiovascular prognosis of "masked hypertension" detected by blood pressure self-measurement in elderly treated hypertensive patients. JAMA. 2004;291:1342–9.
16. Asayama K, Ohkubo T, Metoki H, Obara T, Inoue R, Kikuya M, et al. Cardiovascular outcomes in the first trial of antihypertensive therapy guided by self-measured home blood pressure. Hypertens Res. 2012;35:1102–10.
17. Asayama K. Observational study and participant-level meta-analysis on antihypertensive drug treatment-related cardiovascular risk. Hypertens Res. 2017;40:856–60.
18. Kario K, Saito I, Kushiro T, Teramukai S, Ishikawa Y, Mori Y, et al. Home blood pressure and cardiovascular outcomes in patients during antihypertensive therapy: primary results of HONEST, a large-scale prospective, real-world observational study. Hypertension. 2014;64:989–96.

19. Hoshide S, Yano Y, Haimoto H, Yamagiwa K, Uchiba K, Nagasaka S, et al. Morning and evening home blood pressure and risks of incident stroke and coronary artery disease in the Japanese general practice population: the Japan morning surge-home blood pressure study. Hypertension. 2016;68:54–61.
20. Fujiwara T, Yano Y, Hoshide S, Kanegae H, Kario K. Association of cardiovascular outcomes with masked hypertension defined by home blood pressure monitoring in a Japanese general practice population. JAMA Cardiol. 2018;3:583–90.
21. Niiranen TJ, Asayama K, Thijs L, Johansson JK, Ohkubo T, Kikuya M, et al. Outcome-driven thresholds for home blood pressure measurement: international database of home blood pressure in relation to cardiovascular outcome. Hypertension. 2013;61:27–34.
22. Williams B, Mancia G, Spiering W, Agabiti Rosei E, Azizi M, Burnier M, et al. ESC Scientific Document Group. 2018 ESC/ESH guidelines for the management of arterial hypertension. Eur Heart J. 2018;39:3021–104.
23. Shimamoto K, Ando K, Fujita T, Hasebe N, Higaki J, Horiuchi M, et al. The Japanese Society of Hypertension Guidelines for the Management of Hypertension (JSH 2014). Hypertens Res. 2014;37:253–390.
24. Asayama K, Thijs L, Brguljan-Hitij J, Niiranen TJ, Hozawa A, Boggia J, et al. Risk stratification by self-measured home blood pressure across categories of conventional blood pressure: a participant-level meta-analysis. PLoS Med. 2014;11:e1001591.
25. Nomura K, Asayama K, Thijs L, Niiranen TJ, Lujambio I, Boggia J, et al. Thresholds for conventional and home blood pressure by sex and age in 5018 participants from 5 populations. Hypertension. 2014;64:695–701.
26. Aparicio LS, Thijs L, Boggia J, Jacobs L, Barochiner J, Odili AN, et al. Defining thresholds for home blood pressure monitoring in octogenarians. Hypertension. 2015;66:865–73.
27. Hanazawa T, Asayama K, Watabe D, Tanabe A, Satoh M, Inoue R, et al. Association between amplitude of seasonal variation in self-measured home blood pressure and cardiovascular outcomes: HOMED-BP (hypertension objective treatment based on measurement by electrical devices of blood pressure) study. J Am Heart Assoc. 2018;7:e008509.
28. Matsumoto A, Satoh M, Kikuya M, Ohkubo T, Hirano M, Inoue R, et al. Day-to-day variability in home blood pressure is associated with cognitive decline: the Ohasama study. Hypertension. 2014;63:1333–8.
29. Oishi E, Ohara T, Sakata S, Fukuhara M, Hata J, Yoshida D, et al. Day-to-day blood pressure variability and risk of dementia in a general Japanese elderly population: the Hisayama study. Circulation. 2017;136:516–25.

Diagnostic Value of Home Blood Pressure

5

Kazuomi Kario, Yutaka Imai, Anastasios Kollias, Teemu J. Niiranen, Takayoshi Ohkubo, Richard J. McManus, and George S. Stergiou

K. Kario (✉)
Division of Cardiovascular Medicine, Department of Medicine, Jichi Medical University School of Medicine (JMU), Tochigi, Japan
e-mail: kkario@jichi.ac.jp

Y. Imai
Tohoku Institute for Management of Blood Pressure, Sendai, Japan
e-mail: yutaka.imai.d6@tohoku.ac.jp

A. Kollias · G. S. Stergiou
Hypertension Center STRIDE-7, National and Kapodistrian University of Athens, School of Medicine, Third Department of Medicine, Sotiria Hospital, Athens, Greece
e-mail: gstergi@med.uoa.gr

T. J. Niiranen
Department of Public Health Solutions, National Institute for Health and Welfare, Turku, Finland

Department of Medicine, Turku University Hospital and University of Turku, Turku, Finland
e-mail: teemu.niiranen@thl.fi

T. Ohkubo
Department of Hygiene and Public Health, Teikyo University School of Medicine, Tokyo, Japan

Tohoku Institute for Management of Blood Pressure, Sendai, Japan
e-mail: tohkubo@med.teikyo-u.ac.jp

R. J. McManus
Nuffield Department of Primary Care Health Sciences, University of Oxford, Radcliffe Observatory Quarter, Oxford, UK
e-mail: richard.mcmanus@phc.ox.ac.uk

5.1   Introduction

Recently, new guidelines for the management of hypertension have been released by the European Society of Cardiology/European Society of Hypertension (2018 ESC/ESH guidelines) and American Heart Association/American College of Cardiology (2017 ACC/AHA guidelines) [1, 2]. These guidelines have stressed the importance of out-of-office BPs rather than office BP. There has been a similar emphasis on out-of-office BP-guided management of hypertension in Japan and Asian countries [3–5]. Ambulatory BP monitoring (ABPM) and home BP monitoring (HBPM) are the two standard measurements of out-of-office BPs, and both approaches can detect masked (uncontrolled) hypertension (normotension in office BP and hypertension in out-of-office BP), which carries the highest risk of cardiovascular events, and rule out white-coat hypertension (hypertension in office BP and normotension in out-of-office BP) [1–8].

In current clinical practice, out-of-office BP has been widely accepted as the most accurate modality for the diagnosis and management of hypertension, particularly masked hypertension [6–8]. ABPM is the gold standard, for the diagnosis of masked hypertension. On the other hand, HBPM is also widely used in clinical practice due to its greater practicality, and it can also identify white-coat hypertension and masked hypertension.

5.2   Diagnostic Value of HBPM vs. Office BP Measurement

Previous studies have clearly demonstrated that HBPM has a greater diagnostic value for hypertension than office BP measurement by taking ABPM as reference [9]. HBPM can identify out-of-office hypertension, which is associated with cardiovascular risk, without reference to office BP measurements.

The results of the three measures of BP—i.e., office BP, HBPM, and ABPM—are not always in agreement. For example, Table 5.1 shows the corresponding values of clinic, home, daytime, nighttime, and 24-h BP measurements [2]. The diagnostic BP thresholds of hypertension are 140/90 mmHg for office BP and 135/85 mmHg for home BP. The home BP and daytime ambulatory BP thresholds are comparable, and are 5 mmHg lower than the office BP threshold. At around the 130/80 mmHg level, the office, home, and daytime ambulatory BP levels are correspondent. The difference in BP between the office and out-of-office measures thus becomes more pronounced at the higher BP levels (Table 5.1). This means that the

Table 5.1 Corresponding values of office, home, daytime, nighttime, and 24-h blood pressure measurements

Office	HBPM	Daytime ABPM	Nighttime ABPM	24-h ABPM
120/80	120/80	120/80	100/65	115/75
130/80	130/80	130/80	110/65	125/75
140/90	135/85	135/85	120/70	130/80
160/100	145/90	145/90	140/85	145/90

ABPM ambulatory blood pressure monitoring, *HBPM* home blood pressure monitoring

white-coat effect on BP (office minus out-of-office BP) caused by specific conditions in the office is greater than the difference in the pressor effect between HBPM, measured at rest condition, and ABPM, measured under ambulatory conditions.

The 2017 ACC/AHA guidelines lowered the American diagnostic thresholds for hypertension to 130/80 mmHg both for office and for home BPs [2]. The core concept in these guidelines is the recommendation of earlier and stricter BP control over 24 h, which aims to provide more thorough organ protection and prevent cardiovascular events [10]. This new definition in the 2017 ACC/AHA guidelines markedly changes the prevalence of hypertension subtypes. In the J-HOP (Japan Morning Surge-Home Blood Pressure) study, a general practice-based national home BP registry of outpatients with cardiovascular risk factor (79% medicated with antihypertensive drug) [10], the difference between office and morning home BPs decreases until the two BPs are similar at around a BP threshold of 130/80 mmHg (Fig. 5.1). The prevalence of normotension (well-controlled hypertension), white-coat (uncontrolled) hypertension, masked (uncontrolled) hypertension, and sustained (uncontrolled) hypertension are, respectively, changed from 31%, 15%, 19%, 36% by the ESC/ESH 2018 definition (140/90 mmHg for office BP and 135/85 mmHg for home BP) to 14%, 17%, 10%, 58% by the 2017 ACC/AHA definition (130/80 mmHg for both office and home BPs) (Fig. 5.1) [10]. The population-based Ohasama study also demonstrated the similar change in the distribution of these four classifications [11]. In medicated patients, the prevalence of uncontrolled sustained hypertension is increased, while that of masked uncontrolled hypertension is decreased [10, 11]. The decrease in masked uncontrolled hypertension and the increase in sustained uncontrolled hypertension would give clinicians the opportunity to treat hypertension in this group of patients known to have heightened cardiovascular risk [8].

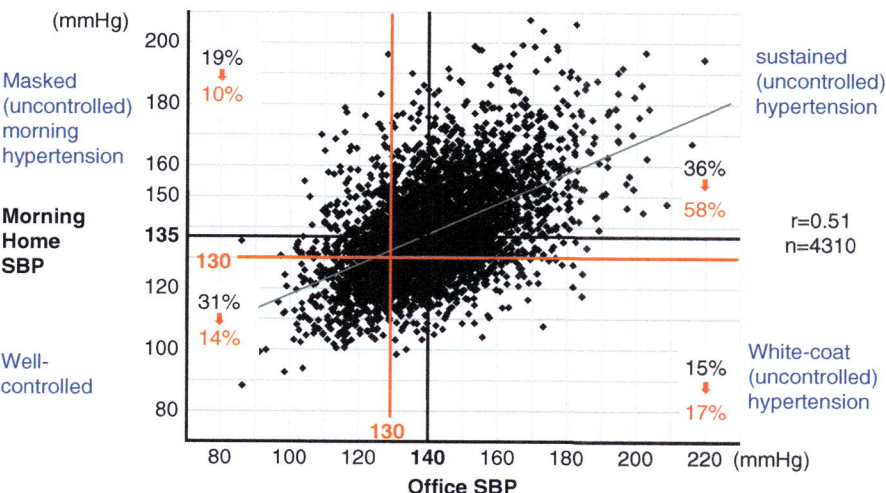

Fig. 5.1 Difference in the prevalence of masked (uncontrolled) hypertension between the 2017 ACC/AHA guidelines (red) and the 2018 ESC/ESH guidelines (black) in subjects in the J-HOP study (Japan Morning Surge-Home Blood Pressure; 4310 medicated hypertensives). *SBP* systolic blood pressure

5.3   Sensitivity and Specificity of HBPM for Diagnosing ABPM-Based Diagnosis of Hypertension

The diagnostic agreement between home and ambulatory BP measurements is a challenging clinical issue. Because the out-of-office BP measurement conditions differ between home BP monitoring and ABPM, the prevalence and characteristics of white-coat hypertension and masked hypertension diagnosed by these two types of monitoring are also different. The main application of HBPM is for the long-term follow-up of treated hypertension. The need for BP assessment out of the office in all treated hypertensive patients is strongly supported by the fact that the white-coat and the masked hypertension phenomena are common in these patients, and the diagnostic value of home BP is as good as in untreated subjects.

Stergiou et al. conducted an extensive systematic review of the use of HBPM for the diagnosis and treatment of hypertension (PubMed, Cochrane Library, 1970–2010) [9, 12, 13]. Sixteen studies of untreated and treated subjects assessed the diagnostic ability of HBPM by taking ABPM as reference. The studies reviewed consistently showed moderate diagnostic agreement between HBPM and ABPM, and superiority of HBPM compared to office measurements in diagnosing uncontrolled hypertension. The diagnostic performance of home BP appeared to be similar across the different populations included in the studies [9, 12, 13]. However, the results on the usefulness of HBPM for the diagnosis of white-coat and masked hypertension were not entirely consistent.

Recently, by using the data of the China Ambulatory and Home BP Registry (N = 1774), which provides the largest number of patients who had undergone ABPM and HBPM within a short period, an accuracy of HBPM in the diagnosis of white-coat and masked hypertension compared to ABPM was tested [14]. This is also the most reliable data using the validated HBPM device, which stores in its BP measurements in memory, and measured by a standardized protocol for 7 consecutive days. In the study, white-coat hypertension is defined as an elevated office BP ($\geq$140/90 mmHg) and a low 24-h ambulatory BP (<130/80 mmHg) or home BPs (<135/85 mmHg), and masked hypertension is defined as a low office BP (<140/90 mmHg) and an elevated 24-h ambulatory BP ($\geq$130/80 mmHg) or home BPs ($\geq$135/85 mmHg). In untreated patients (n = 573), the prevalence of white-coat hypertension (13.1% vs. 19.9%), masked hypertension (17.8% vs. 13.1%), and sustained hypertension (46.4% vs. 39.6%) were significantly ($P < 0.02$) different between 24-h ABPM and HBPM. In treated patients (n = 1201), only the prevalence of masked hypertension differed significantly (18.7% vs. 14.5%; $P < 0.005$) (Table 5.2). Regardless of the treatment status, home BP compared with 24-h ambulatory BP had low sensitivity (range 47–74%), but high specificity (86–94%), and accordingly low positive (41–87%), but high negative predictive values (80–94%), and had moderate diagnostic agreement (82–85%) and Kappa statistic (0.41–0.66). Thus, HBPM has high specificity, but low sensitivity in the diagnosis of white-coat and masked hypertension, and may therefore behave as a complement to, but not a replacement of, ABPM.

Table 5.2 Diagnostic accuracy of home vs. 24-h ambulatory blood pressure monitoring in treated ($n = 1201$) and untreated patients ($n = 573$)

Treatment status and hypertension subtype	Sensitivity (%)	Specificity (%)	Positive predictive value (%)	Negative predictive value (%)	Agreement (%)	Kappa statistic
Treated patients						
Uncontrolled clinic pressure and controlled ambulatory or home pressure	52 (46–59)	89 (87–91)	53 (47–60)	88 (86–90)	82	0.41*
Masked uncontrolled hypertension	47 (41–54)	93 (91–95)	61 (54–68)	88 (86–90)	84	0.45*
Sustained uncontrolled hypertension	72 (67–77)	86 (84–88)	71 (67–75)	86 (84–89)	82	0.58*
Untreated patients						
White-coat hypertension	62 (51–73)	86 (83–89)	41 (32–50)	94 (91–96)	83	0.40*
Masked hypertension	47 (37–56)	94 (92–96)	64 (53–74)	89 (86–91)	85	0.46*
Sustained hypertension	74 (69–80)	90 (87–94)	87 (83–92)	80 (76–85)	83	0.66*

Values in the parentheses are 95% confidence interval.
*$P < 0.0001$.

Kang YY, et al. J Hypertens 2015; 33: 1580–7

A recent cross-sectional study of a multiethnic population of 551 participants (age, 40–75 years; 246 white British, 147 South Asian and 158 African Caribbean subjects) with and without a previous diagnosis of hypertension recruited from 28 primary care practices compared the test performance of clinic BP (using various protocols) and HBPM (1 week) with a reference standard of mean daytime ambulatory measurements using a threshold of 140/90 mmHg for office and 135/85 mmHg for out-of-office measurement [15]. For people without hypertension, office measurement using three different methodologies had high specificity (75–97%) but variable sensitivity (33–65%), whereas HBPM had a sensitivity of 68–88% and specificity of 64–80%, indicating that ABPM remains a better choice for diagnosing hypertension compared to the other modes of BP measurement regardless of ethnicity. For people with hypertension, the use of office measurements for the detection of elevated BP had a sensitivity of 34–69% and specificity of 73–92%, while the use of HBPM had a sensitivity of 81–88% and specificity of 55–65%. Differences in the accuracy of HBPM and office BP measurement (higher sensitivity of the former; higher specificity of the latter) were also not affected by ethnicity.

In the IDH study (Improving the Detection of Hypertension), which examined the overlap between ABPM and HBPM for the detection of masked hypertension in 333 community-dwelling unmedicated adults with office BP <140/90 mmHg, masked hypertension was defined by the presence of daytime (mean daytime BP ≥135/85 mmHg), 24-h (mean 24-h BP ≥130/80 mmHg), or nighttime (mean nighttime BP ≥120/70 mmHg) hypertension, and home masked hypertension was defined as mean BP ≥135/85 mmHg on HBPM [16]. The prevalence of masked hypertension was 25.8% for ambulatory masked hypertension and 11.1% for home masked hypertension. Among participants with masked hypertension on either ABPM or HBPM, 29.5% had masked hypertension on both ABPM and HBPM; 61.1% had masked hypertension only on ABPM; and 9.4% of participants had masked hypertension only on HBPM. After multivariable adjustment and compared with participants without masked hypertension on ABPM and HBPM, those with masked hypertension on both ABPM and HBPM and only on ABPM had a higher left ventricular mass index (mean difference, 12.7 g/m^2, $P < 0.001$; and 4.9 g/m^2, $P = 0.022$, respectively), whereas participants with masked hypertension only on HBPM did not have an increased left ventricular mass index (mean difference [SE], −1.9 [4.8] g/m^2, $P = 0.693$). Thus, ABPM and HBPM will detect many individuals with masked hypertension who have an increased cardiovascular disease risk [17].

When using the BP thresholds recommended in the 2017 ACC/AHA guidelines, the prevalence of ambulatory masked hypertension, daytime masked hypertension, 24-h masked hypertension, nighttime masked hypertension, and home masked hypertension were 40.6%, 21.8%, 25.6%, 32.1%, and 16.2%, respectively [16]. A higher percentage of participants had masked hypertension only on ABPM and masked hypertension on both ABPM and HBPM compared with the percentages when using the BP thresholds from the primary analysis. The prevalence of partial masked hypertension on either HBPM or ABPM and sustained hypertension on both ABPM and HBPM were 10.4% and 22.7%, respectively, in the Ohasama study [11].

These findings on the diagnostic agreement of HBPM with ABPM should take into account the imperfect reproducibility of the two methods, which is responsible for some diagnostic disagreement even if the same method (ABPM or HBPM) is performed twice, and suggest that in fact the diagnostic agreement between the two methods is better than suggested by these studies [13].

5.4   Diagnostic Value for Nocturnal Hypertension

In the past, nighttime BP has been measured by ABPM, but more recently nocturnal HBPM has also been developed for introduction into clinical practice [18–21].

Nocturnal hypertension is frequently found in high-risk patients having diabetes, chronic kidney disease, or sleep apnea, and thus the detection of nocturnal hypertension by ABPM or nocturnal HBPM and the management of uncontrolled nocturnal hypertension might be recommended even in patients with normotension that is well controlled by office and morning home BPs.

Nocturnal hypertension is defined by the threshold of 120/70 mmHg for ABPM. The diagnostic value of HBPM for nocturnal hypertension is not well established. However, several papers have demonstrated that nocturnal HBPM is valuable for the diagnosis of nocturnal hypertension diagnosed by ABPM. In our J-HOP study (N = 854), nighttime home systolic BP (the average of nighttime BPs measured automatically at 2:00, 3:00, and 4:00 am) was slightly higher than nighttime ambulatory systolic BP (difference, 2.6 mmHg; $P < 0.001$) [22]. A two-night home BP schedule (six readings) appears to be the minimum requirement for a reliable assessment of nighttime home BP—i.e., an assessment that shows reasonable agreement with ambulatory BP and reasonable association with the observed preclinical organ damage [23]. In a crossover study using information and communication technology (ICT)-based nocturnal HBPM, the reliability of nocturnal HBPM appeared to be similar whether the HBPM was adapted to the chosen bedtime of participants (measurement at 2, 3, and 4 h after a chosen bedtime) or measured at fixed time points (2:00, 3:00, and 4:00 am) [24].

The standard threshold to diagnose nocturnal hypertension using nighttime ambulatory BP is ≥120/70 mmHg. The 2017 ACC/AHA guidelines defined a threshold of nocturnal BP (110/65 mmHg) corresponding to clinic, home, and daytime BPs (all 130/80 mmHg) (Table 5.1). There are no guidelines on how to measure nocturnal HBPM (how many measurements on how many nights) and what the thresholds for nocturnal home hypertension should be. The J-HOP study, which is the first clinic-based prospective study using nocturnal HBPM, demonstrated that even after controlling morning BP, a risk of uncontrolled nocturnal hypertension remains [25]. The new criteria for nighttime BP threshold from the 2017 ACC/AHA guidelines might not contribute to a reduction in masked uncontrolled hypertension. A morning home systolic BP of 135 mmHg corresponds to a nighttime home systolic BP of 120 mmHg, which is the threshold defined by the Seventh Report of the Joint National Committee on Prevention, while the 110 mmHg threshold of the 2017 ACC/AHA guidelines corresponds to a morning home systolic BP of

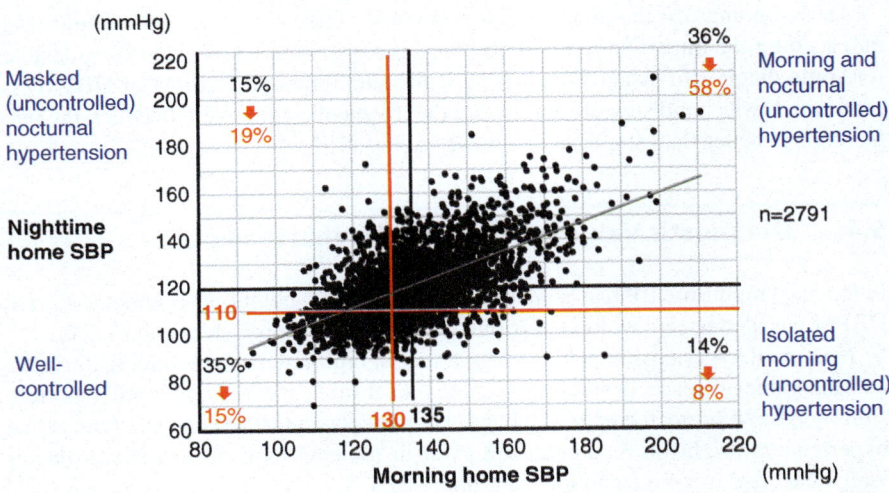

Fig. 5.2 Difference in the prevalence of nocturnal (uncontrolled) hypertension between the 2017 ACC/AHA guidelines (red) and the 2018 ESH/ECC guidelines (black) in subjects in the J-HOP study (Japan Morning Surge-Home Blood Pressure; 2791 medicated hypertensives). SBP, systolic blood pressure

130 mmHg. In those with well-controlled morning home systolic BP, a significant proportion of patients continue to have uncontrolled nocturnal hypertension (30% by the criteria of 135 mmHg for morning home systolic BP and 120 mmHg for nighttime SBP; 56% by the criteria of 130 mmHg for morning home systolic BP and 110 mmHg for nighttime SBP) (Fig. 5.2) [25]. Thus, to detect the residual risk of uncontrolled nocturnal hypertension, nocturnal HBPM would be recommended even in patients with well-controlled normotension based on clinic BP and/or morning home BPs.

5.5   Clinical Benefit of HBPM-Based Diagnosis of Hypertension

The most important diagnostic advantages of HBPM are that it employs a higher number of BP readings by repeated self-measurement compared to an office visit and that these are taken in the usual environment of which individual. To minimize the cardiovascular risk associated with raised blood pressure, uncontrolled hypertension should be controlled to below the target BP levels as soon as possible. Out-of-office BP is not stable, and it changes with various day-by-day personal and environmental conditions such as seasonal variation. By the real-world stress at that time, hypertension may be developed silently before visiting doctor's office. Ideally, self-measured HBPM should support the diagnosis of out-of-office hypertension without the characteristic delay of diagnoses based on the office and/or ABPM.

References

1. Williams B, Mancia G, Spiering W, Agabiti Rosei E, Azizi M, Burnier M, et al. 2018 ESC/ESH guidelines for the management of arterial hypertension. Eur Heart J. 2018;39:3021–104.
2. Whelton PK, Carey RM, Aronow WS, Casey DE Jr, Collins KJ, Dennison Himmelfarb C, et al. 2017 ACC/AHA/AAPA/ABC/ACPM/AGS/APhA/ASH/ASPC/NMA/PCNA guideline for the prevention, detection, evaluation, and Management of High Blood Pressure in adults: executive summary: a report of the American College of Cardiology/American Heart Association task force on clinical practice guidelines. Hypertension. 2018;71:1269–324.
3. Shimamoto K, Ando K, Fujita T, Hasebe N, Higaki J, Horiuchi M, et al. The Japanese Society of Hypertension Guidelines for the Management of Hypertension (JSH 2014). Hypertens Res. 2014;37:253–390.
4. Park S, Buranakitjaroen P, Chen CH, Chia YC, Divinagracia R, Hoshide S, et al. Expert panel consensus recommendations for home blood pressure monitoring in Asia: the Hope Asia network. J Hum Hypertens. 2018;32:249–58.
5. Kario K, Park S, Buranakitjaroen P, Chia YC, Chen CH, Divinagracia R, et al. Guidance on home blood pressure monitoring: a statement of the HOPE Asia Network. J Clin Hypertens. 2018;20:456–61.
6. Pierdomenico SD, Pierdomenico AM, Coccina F, Clement DL, De Buyzere ML, De Bacquer DA, et al. Prognostic value of masked uncontrolled hypertension. Hypertension. 2018;72:862–9.
7. Kario K, Thijs L, Staessen JA. Blood pressure measurement and treatment decisions: masked and white coat hypertension. Circ Res. 2019;124(7):990–1008.
8. Banegas JR, Ruilope LM, de la Sierra A, Vinyoles E, Gorostidi M, de la Cruz JJ, et al. Relationship between clinic and ambulatory blood-pressure measurements and mortality. N Engl J Med. 2018;378:1509–20.
9. Stergiou GS, Bliziotis IA. Home blood pressure monitoring in the diagnosis and treatment of hypertension: a systematic review. Am J Hypertens. 2011;24:123–34.
10. Kario K. Global impact of 2017 American Heart Association/American College of Cardiology Hypertension Guidelines: a perspective from Japan. Circulation. 2018;137:543–5.
11. Satoh M, Asayama K, Murakami T, Kikuya M, Metoki H, Imai Y, et al. Stroke risk due to partial white-coat or masked hypertension based on the ACC/AHA guideline's blood pressure threshold: the Ohasama study. Hypertens Res. 2019;42:120–2.
12. Stergiou GS, Kollias A, Zeniodi M, Karpettas N, Ntineri A. Home blood pressure monitoring: primary role in hypertension management. Curr Hypertens Rep. 2014;16(8):462.
13. Stergiou GS, Ntineri A. The optimal schedule for self-home blood pressure monitoring. J Hypertens. 2015;33(4):693–7.
14. Kang YY, Li Y, Huang QF, Song J, Shan XL, Dou Y, Xu XJ, Chen SH, Wang JG. Accuracy of home versus ambulatory blood pressure monitoring in the diagnosis of white-coat and masked hypertension. J Hypertens. 2015;33:1580–7.
15. Gill P, Haque MS, Martin U, Mant J, Mohammed MA, Heer G, et al. Measurement of blood pressure for the diagnosis and management of hypertension in different ethnic groups: one size fits all. BMC Cardiovasc Disord. 2017;17:55.
16. Anstey DE, Muntner P, Bello NA, Pugliese DN, Yano Y, Kronish IM, et al. Diagnosing masked hypertension using ambulatory blood pressure monitoring, home blood pressure monitoring, or both? Hypertension. 2018;72:1200–7.
17. Satoh M, Asayama K, Kikuya M, Inoue R, Metoki H, Hosaka M, et al. Long-term stroke risk due to partial white-coat or masked hypertension based on home and ambulatory blood pressure measurements: the Ohasama study. Hypertension. 2016;67:48–55.
18. Andreadis EA, Agaliotis G, Kollias A, Kolyvas G, Achimastos A, Stergiou GS. Night-time home versus ambulatory blood pressure in determining target organ damage. J Hypertens. 2016;34:438–44.

19. Kario K. Nocturnal hypertension: new technology and evidence. Hypertension. 2018;71:997–1009.
20. Asayama K, Fujiwara T, Hoshide S, Ohkubo T, Kario K, Stergiou GS, et al. Nocturnal blood pressure measured by home devices: evidence and perspective for clinical application. J Hypertens. 2019;37(5):905–16.
21. Imai Y, Asayama K, Fujiwara S, Saito K, Sato H, Haga T, et al. Development and evaluation of a home nocturnal blood pressure monitoring system using a wrist-cuff device. Blood Press Monit. 2018;23:318–26.
22. Ishikawa J, Hoshide S, Eguchi K, Ishikawa S, Shimada K, Kario K, et al. Nighttime home blood pressure and the risk of hypertensive target organ damage. Hypertension. 2012;60:921–8.
23. Kollias A, Andreadis E, Agaliotis G, Kolyvas GN, Achimastos A, Stergiou GS. The optimal night-time home blood pressure monitoring schedule: agreement with ambulatory blood pressure and association with organ damage. J Hypertens. 2018;36:243–9.
24. Fujiwara T, Nishizawa M, Hoshide S, Kanegae H, Kario K. Comparison of different schedules of nocturnal home blood pressure measurement using an information/communication technology-based device in hypertensive patients. J Clin Hypertens. 2018;20:1633–41.
25. Kario K, Wang JG. Could 130/80 mm hg be adopted as the diagnostic threshold and management goal of hypertension in consideration of the characteristics of Asian populations? Hypertension. 2018;71:979–84.

Home Blood Pressure Monitoring Schedule

6

Teemu J. Niiranen, Richard J. McManus,
Takayoshi Ohkubo, and George S. Stergiou

6.1   Introduction

The optimal schedule for performing the home blood pressure measurements is still debated. If a standard home blood pressure measurement protocol is not always used, correct interpretation of home readings may be challenging in both clinical and research settings. Several factors need to be considered when trying to define an optimal home blood pressure measurement schedule: i) the number of measurement days; ii) the time of day and day of the week of blood pressure measurement; iii) the number of measurements performed on one measurement occasion; iv) the interval

T. J. Niiranen (✉)
Department of Public Health Solutions, National Institute for Health and Welfare,
Turku, Finland

Department of Medicine, Turku University Hospital and University of Turku,
Turku, Finland
e-mail: teemu.niiranen@thl.fi

R. J. McManus
Nuffield Department of Primary Care Health Sciences, University of Oxford,
Radcliffe Observatory Quarter, Oxford, UK
e-mail: richard.mcmanus@phc.ox.ac.uk

T. Ohkubo
Department of Hygiene and Public Health, Teikyo University School of Medicine,
Tokyo, Japan

Tohoku Institute for Management of Blood Pressure, Sendai, Japan
e-mail: tohkubo@med.teikyo-u.ac.jp

G. S. Stergiou
Hypertension Center STRIDE-7, National and Kapodistrian University of Athens, School of Medicine, Third Department of Medicine, Sotiria Hospital, Athens, Greece
e-mail: gstergi@med.uoa.gr

© The Editor(s), under exclusive license to Springer Nature Switzerland AG 2020
G. S. Stergiou et al. (eds.), *Home Blood Pressure Monitoring*,
Updates in Hypertension and Cardiovascular Protection,
https://doi.org/10.1007/978-3-030-23065-4_6

55

between successive measurements; and v) the need to exclude readings of certain measurement days. This chapter describes the up-to-date research for the optimal protocol of home blood pressure measurement and the differences in measurement protocols recommended by various international hypertension guidelines.

6.2   Cross-Sectional Studies

Several population studies have demonstrated that home blood pressure level and variability decrease slowly with the number of measurements as the patients become more accustomed to measuring their blood pressure [1–3]. It is therefore conceivable that the lower and more stable readings obtained at the end of the measurement period could represent the patient's "true" blood pressure more accurately than the initial readings. Before prospective data became available, numerous cross-sectional studies assessed the optimal number of home blood pressure measurements in samples of hypertensive patients. These studies mainly focused on finding a statistical "sweet spot" for the number of measurements, over which the reproducibility of the readings over multiple days would not materially increase anymore. In a study by Chatellier et al., 79 hypertensive patients measured their blood pressure at home thrice in the morning and evening for 21 days [4]. The authors then demonstrated that 80% of the maximal reproducibility (reduction in the standard deviation of differences between the average values of two home blood pressure sessions) was obtained by averaging 15 measurements over the initial 5 days [4]. In another study from the same first author, 1710 hypertensive patients measured their blood pressure three times in the morning and evening over 4 days while discarding the measurements of the first day [5]. When the number of measurements was increased from 1 to 18, the standard deviation of systolic/diastolic mean blood pressure was reduced by 17%/23%. However, 85% of this reduction was already achieved by six measurements taken at random [5]. In two studies with samples of 133 and 189 hypertensive patients, Stergiou et al. demonstrated that at least 12 measurements taken on 3 days are needed for the reproducibility of home blood pressure to be superior to that of conventional measurements [6, 7]. Combined, the results of all these studies suggest that most of the reduction in home blood pressure variability occurs over the initial 6–15 measurements.

Correct blood pressure classification, on which treatment decisions are based, however, often plays a more important role in clinical practice than the statistical reproducibility of measurements. In a sample of 4802 individuals from three populations included in the International Database on HOme blood pressure in relation to Cardiovascular Outcomes (IDHOCO), the participants were divided into groups by their (1) office and home blood pressure (normotension, masked hypertension, white-coat hypertension, and sustained hypertension) and (2) home blood pressure level (normal blood pressure, high normal blood pressure, grade 1 and 2 hypertension), while the number of single home measurements was increased from one to seven [8]. The results of this study demonstrated that agreement in classification between consecutive measurement days indicated near perfect agreement (Cohen's kappa coefficient ≥ 0.9) after the sixth measurement day for both office-home blood pressure cross-classification and home blood pressure level [8].

A third method for assessing the optimal home blood pressure schedule in a cross-sectional setting is to examine the relation between an increasing number of home readings and hypertensive organ damage. In a mixed sample of 464 participants and hypertensive patients, Johansson et al. examined the correlations of home blood pressure with echocardiography and albuminuria [9]. Again, the highest correlations were observed when the mean of all available 28 measurements taken over a period of 7 days was used. However, most of the increase in correlation occurred during the initial 4 days (16 measurements). No significant improvement was observed when the measurements performed on the first day were discarded. Furthermore, morning and evening home blood pressure correlated equally well with signs of organ damage. The results were similar in hypertensive patients and in individuals randomly drawn from the population register [9].

In addition to the number of measurements, a single cross-sectional study has assessed the impact of the day of the week on home blood pressure level and day-to-day blood pressure profile in a population-based sample of 1852 Finns [10]. The authors examined how the initial measurement day of the week affects 3-day and 7-day mean home blood pressure and the blood pressure variation between different days of the week. In this sample, there were no differences in mean blood pressures that were initiated on various days of the week. However, systolic and diastolic blood pressure were slightly (all differences <2 mmHg), but statistically significantly, lower during the weekend than during weekdays. The authors concluded that a 7-day home BP measurement period can be initiated on any given day of the week. However, if measurements are performed on only 3 days, it was recommended to keep in mind that blood pressure is usually the lowest during the weekend, and highest at the beginning of the week, particularly among the employed [10].

A single, small study with 56 patients has also assessed if a shorter 10-s interval would give a better prediction of the average 24-h blood pressure than home blood pressure readings taken at normal 1-min intervals [11]. In this study, however, blood pressure readings taken at 1-min intervals were considerably lower and were significantly closer to mean awake ambulatory blood pressure. No differences in patients' compliance were observed in taking adequate numbers of readings at the different time intervals.

6.3   Prospective Studies

Instead of cross-sectional analyses based on reproducibility, classification, and associations with organ damage, the optimal home blood pressure measurement schedule should preferably be determined based on outcome data. In two large population-based studies from Japan and Finland with somewhat different measurement protocols (single measurements in the morning and evening for up to 28 days in the Ohasama cohort [n = 1491], duplicate measurements in the morning and evening for 7 days in the Finn-Home cohort [n = 2081]), the prognostic value of home blood pressure for cardiovascular disease increased only slightly within the range of 1–7 days (Fig. 6.1) [12, 13]. Although no statistically significant differences in the hazard ratios were observed, the majority of the steady increase in risk occurred during the first 3–4 days (Fig. 6.1). The results of a Greek study with a

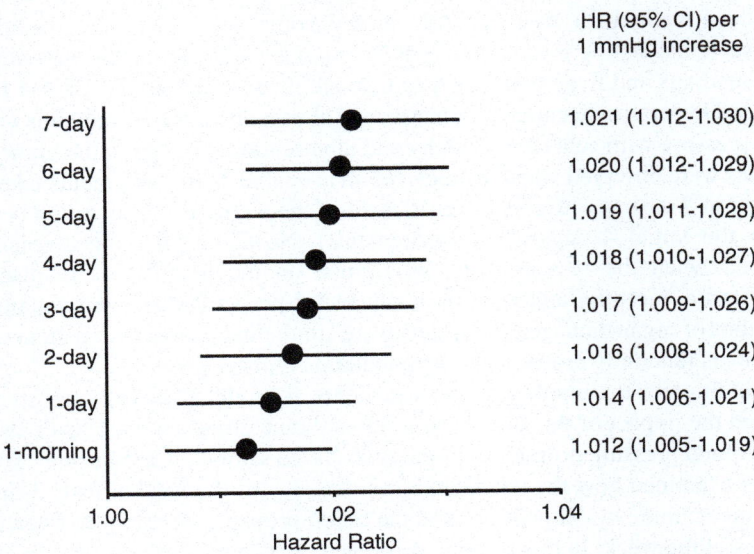

Fig. 6.1 Association of systolic home blood pressure and incident cardiovascular disease on cumulative days of home measurement in the Finn-Home Study. Duplicate measurements in the morning and evening were performed on each measurement day [12] *HR* hazard ratio, *CI* confidence interval

population sample of 662 individuals provided similar results—the predictive power of home blood pressure increased only slightly as the number of measurements increased from 1 to 12 over a period of 3 days [14]. Another analysis based on the first seven morning measurements of the Finn-Home, Ohasama, and Tsurugaya cohorts (n = 4802; IDHOCO consortium) demonstrated that although the hazard ratios for cardiovascular disease increase with the number of measurements, the confidence intervals were too wide and overlapping to show superiority of multiple measurement days over the first measurement day [8]. Indeed, the majority of the predictive power of home blood pressure is obtained already on the first measurement day (Fig. 6.1) [12–15].

The Finn-Home investigators have also performed in-depth analyses in which they observed that (1) no additional benefit in predictive ability for cardiovascular disease is achieved when the values obtained during the first day of measurement are discarded when calculating the mean blood pressure based on 7 days; (2) morning and evening blood pressure are equally predictive; and (3) measurement of home blood pressure twice, instead of once, on each measurement occasion offers a marginally better predictive value as it naturally doubles the number of measurements [12]. These observations were made using data based on duplicate measurements performed in the morning and evening over seven days. Although morning and evening blood pressure seem to have an equally good predictive value, blood pressure measurement in the morning and evening is still justifiable in treated patients to determine 24-hour drug efficacy [16, 17]. In addition, exclusion of the first measurement day could have an effect if measurements are performed on only three measurement days, instead of seven.

Studies on the optimal schedule of home blood pressure measurement for assessing blood pressure variability are scarce. In a 2008 article, Kikuya et al. briefly mention in that ten home measurements could be sufficient for estimating blood pressure variability in the Ohasama study sample [18]. This suggestion was, however, based solely on the observations of a 10-day standard deviation of home blood pressure being similar to a 30-day home blood pressure standard deviation in a sample of 157 individuals. In a prospective study based on the Finn-Home cohort data ($n = 1706$), blood pressure variability of the mean of two morning systolic blood pressure measurements on 3 days was related to incident cardiovascular disease, with hazard ratios increasing only marginally thereafter [19].

6.3.1   Recommendations of the Current Hypertension Guidelines

In contrast to earlier recommendations, the recommendations of the current international hypertension guidelines on the schedule of home blood pressure measurement are relatively similar (Table 6.1) [20–23]. However, one must remember that although the differences between guidelines have decreased, physicians' and patients' adherence to the recommendations of these guidelines remains nevertheless suboptimal [24, 25].

All major guidelines currently recommend duplicate measurements on each measurement occasion in the morning and evening. Only the British guidelines still recommend discarding the first measurement day whereas this recommendation was removed from the most recent 2018 European hypertension guidelines [20, 22]. The guidelines also in general agree on the number of measurement days (Table 6.1). Only the American guidelines are markedly different from the others in this aspect as they recommend daily measurements in an ideal situation, whereas weekly measurements are also acceptable [23].

These recommendations are mainly meant for short-term use, i.e., for diagnosing hypertension, before visits to the doctor's office, or when antihypertensive treatment has been changed. For long-term follow-up of hypertension, a different

Table 6.1 Home blood pressure measurement schedules recommended by various guidelines

Guideline	Number of measurements on each occasion	Number of days	Morning and evening measurements	Discard first day
European [20]	2	At least 3, preferably 7	Yes	No
American [23]	≥2	Optimally daily; ideally 7	Yes	No
Japanese [21]	2	≥5	Yes	No
British [22]	2	At least 4, ideally 7	Yes	Yes

schedule is needed. However, evidence to support such a schedule is scarce. The European Society of Hypertension 2010 home blood pressure measurement guidelines, for example, recommend "less frequent measurements, for example, once or twice per week" for long-term follow-up of blood pressure at home [26].

Patients' views also have a bearing on the feasibility of monitoring schedules. In one focus group based qualitative study in the United Kingdom, patients described preferring both shorter and more flexible schedules over and above the more rigid twice daily for 7 days regime commonly recommended at that time [27].

6.4   Conclusions

In general, the current literature suggests that the predictive accuracy of home blood pressure increases with the number of measurements without a clear threshold. It is therefore likely that the number of measurements is the most important factor in home blood pressure accuracy [28]. Unfortunately, the number of recommended home measurements is a double-edged sword. Although a longer measurement period will always slightly increase diagnostic accuracy, the probability of lower compliance and errors in a generalized use increases at the same time. The existing data suggest that most of the benefit in increased accuracy is achieved already during the initial three to four measurement days when duplicate measurements are performed in the morning and evening. No good evidence exists that measurements performed on the first day of measurements need to be discarded, particularly when 7 days of measurements are used. Despite preliminary findings, more research is warranted on the optimal interval between successive measurements, on the impact of the day of the week on home blood pressure, and the optimal schedule for assessing home blood pressure variability. Although the recommendations of the current hypertension guidelines on the schedule of home blood pressure measurement (duplicate measurements in the morning and evening on ≥ 3 days) agree relatively well with each other and the literature, additional research and collaboration is needed to create a uniform international recommendation on the optimal schedule of home blood pressure measurement.

References

1. Niiranen TJ, Jula AM, Kantola IM, Reunanen A. Comparison of agreement between clinic and home-measured blood pressure in the Finnish population: the Finn-HOME Study. J Hypertens. 2006;24(8):1549–55.
2. Stergiou GS, Skeva I, Baibas NM, Kalkana CB, Roussias LG, Mountokalakis TD. Diagnosis of hypertension using home or ambulatory blood pressure monitoring: comparison with the conventional strategy based on repeated clinic blood pressure measurements. J Hypertens. 2000;18(12):1745–51.
3. Hond ED, Celis H, Fagard R, Keary L, Leeman M, O'Brien E, et al. Self-measured versus ambulatory blood pressure in the diagnosis of hypertension. J Hypertens. 2003;21(4):717–22.
4. Chatellier G, Day M, Bobrie G, Menard J. Feasibility study of N-of-1 trials with blood pressure self-monitoring in hypertension. Hypertension. 1995;25(2):294–301.

5. Chatellier G, Dutrey-Dupagne C, Vaur L, Zannad F, Genes N, Elkik F, et al. Home self blood pressure measurement in general practice. The SMART study. Self-measurement for the Assessment of the Response to Trandolapril. Am J Hypertens. 1996;9(7):644–52.
6. Stergiou GS, Skeva I, Zourbaki AS, Mountokalakis TD. Self-monitoring of blood pressure at home: how many measurements are needed? J Hypertens. 1998;16(6):725–31.
7. Stergiou GS, Baibas NM, Gantzarou AP, Skeva II, Kalkana CB, Roussias LG, et al. Reproducibility of home, ambulatory, and clinic blood pressure: implications for the design of trials for the assessment of antihypertensive drug efficacy. Am J Hypertens. 2002;15(2):101–4.
8. Niiranen TJ, Asayama K, Thijs L, Johansson JK, Hara A, Hozawa A, et al. Optimal number of days for home blood pressure measurement. Am J Hypertens. 2015;28(5):595–603.
9. Johansson JK, Niiranen TJ, Puukka PJ, Jula AM. Optimal schedule for home blood pressure monitoring based on a clinical approach. J Hypertens. 2010;28(2):259–64.
10. Juhanoja EP, Puukka PJ, Johansson JK, Niiranen TJ, Jula AM. The impact of the day of the week on home blood pressure: the Finn-Home study. Blood Press Monit. 2016;21(2):63–8.
11. Eguchi K, Kuruvilla S, Ogedegbe G, Gerin W, Schwartz JE, Pickering TG. What is the optimal interval between successive home blood pressure readings using an automated oscillometric device? J Hypertens. 2009;27(6):1172–7.
12. Niiranen TJ, Johansson JK, Reunanen A, Jula AM. Optimal schedule for home blood pressure measurement based on prognostic data: the Finn-Home Study. Hypertension. 2011;57(6):1081–6.
13. Ohkubo T, Asayama K, Kikuya M, Metoki H, Hoshi H, Hashimoto J, et al. How many times should blood pressure be measured at home for better prediction of stroke risk? Ten-year follow-up results from the Ohasama study. J Hypertens. 2004;22(6):1099–104.
14. Stergiou GS, Nasothimiou EG, Kalogeropoulos PG, Pantazis N, Baibas NM. The optimal home blood pressure monitoring schedule based on the Didima outcome study. J Hum Hypertens. 2010;24(3):158–64.
15. Sega R, Facchetti R, Bombelli M, Cesana G, Corrao G, Grassi G, et al. Prognostic value of ambulatory and home blood pressures compared with office blood pressure in the general population—Follow-up results from the Pressioni Arteriose Monitorate e Loro Associazioni (PAMELA) study. Circulation. 2005;111(14):1777–83.
16. Zannad F, Vaur L, Dutrey-Dupagne C, Genes N, Chatellier G, Elkik F, et al. Assessment of drug efficacy using home self-blood pressure measurement: the SMART study. Self measurement for the assessment of the response to Trandolapril. J Hum Hypertens. 1996;10(6):341–7.
17. Stergiou GS, Efstathiou SP, Skeva II, Baibas NM, Kalkana CB, Mountokalakis TD. Assessment of drug effects on blood pressure and pulse pressure using clinic, home and ambulatory measurements. J Hum Hypertens. 2002;16(10):729–35.
18. Kikuya M, Ohkubo T, Metoki H, Asayama K, Hara A, Obara T, et al. Day-by-day variability of blood pressure and heart rate at home as a novel predictor of prognosis: the Ohasama study. Hypertension. 2008;52(6):1045–50.
19. Juhanoja EP, Johansson JK, Puukka PJ, Jula AM, Niiranen TJ. Optimal schedule for assessing home BP variability: the Finn-Home Study. Am J Hypertens. 2018;31(6):715–25.
20. Williams B, Mancia G, Spiering W, Agabiti Rosei E, Azizi M, et al. 2018 ESC/ESH guidelines for the management of arterial hypertension: the task force for the management of arterial hypertension of the European Society of Cardiology and the European Society of Hypertension: the task force for the management of arterial hypertension of the European Society of Cardiology and the European Society of Hypertension. J Hypertens. 2018;36(10):1953–2041.
21. Shimamoto K, Ando K, Fujita T, Hasebe N, Higaki J, Horiuchi M, et al. The Japanese Society of Hypertension Guidelines for the Management of Hypertension (JSH 2014). Hypertens Res. 2014;37(4):253–390.
22. Krause T, Lovibond K, Caulfield M, McCormack T, Williams B, Guideline Development G. Management of hypertension: summary of NICE guidance. BMJ. 2011;343:d4891.
23. Shen WK, Sheldon RS, Benditt DG, Cohen MI, Forman DE, Goldberger ZD, et al. 2017 ACC/AHA/HRS guideline for the evaluation and Management of Patients with Syncope: a report of the American College of Cardiology/American Heart Association task force on clinical practice guidelines and the Heart Rhythm Society. Circulation. 2017;136(5):e60–e122.

24. Milot JP, Birnbaum L, Larochelle P, Wistaff R, Laskine M, Van Nguyen P, et al. Unreliability of home blood pressure measurement and the effect of a patient-oriented intervention. Can J Cardiol. 2015;31(5):658–63.
25. Ozone S, Sato M, Takayashiki A, Sakamoto N, Yoshimoto H, Maeno T. Adherence to blood pressure measurement guidelines in long-term care facilities: a cross sectional study. J Gen Fam Med. 2018;19(3):97–101.
26. Parati G, Stergiou GS, Asmar R, Bilo G, de Leeuw P, Imai Y, et al. European Society of Hypertension practice guidelines for home blood pressure monitoring. J Hum Hypertens. 2010;24(12):779–85.
27. Grant S, Hodgkinson JA, Milner SL, Martin U, Tompson A, Hobbs FR, et al. Patients' and clinicians' views on the optimum schedules for self-monitoring of blood pressure: a qualitative focus group and interview study. Br J Gen Pract. 2016;66(652):e819–e30.
28. Brook RD. Home blood pressure: accuracy is independent of monitoring schedules. Am J Hypertens. 2000;13(6 Pt 1):625–31.

Home Blood Pressure Monitoring for Treatment Titration

7

Richard J. McManus, Jonathan Mant, Takayoshi Ohkubo, Yutaka Imai, and Kazuomi Kario

7.1 Background

Since the first trials of antihypertensives in the 1960s, the management of hypertension has involved the titration of blood pressure against dose of treatment [1]. The Structured care and Hypertension Detection and Follow up (HDFP) trial showed that structured care with regular titration against clinic blood pressure not only led

R. J. McManus (✉)
Nuffield Department of Primary Care Health Sciences, University of Oxford,
Radcliffe Observatory Quarter, Oxford, UK
e-mail: richard.mcmanus@phc.ox.ac.uk

J. Mant
Primary Care Unit, Strangeways Research Laboratory, Department of Public Health
and Primary Care, University of Cambridge, Cambridge, UK
e-mail: jm677@medschl.cam.ac.uk

T. Ohkubo
Department of Hygiene and Public Health, Teikyo University School of Medicine, Tokyo, Japan

Tohoku Institute for Management of Blood Pressure, Sendai, Japan
e-mail: tohkubo@med.teikyo-u.ac.jp

Y. Imai
Tohoku Institute for Management of Blood Pressure, Sendai, Japan
e-mail: yutaka.imai.d6@tohoku.ac.jp

K. Kario
Division of Cardiovascular Medicine, Department of Medicine, Jichi Medical University
School of Medicine (JMU), Tochigi, Japan
e-mail: kkario@jichi.ac.jp

to lower blood pressure than usual care but also a mortality improvement [2]. There are also data from primary care suggesting that those patients whose BP is titrated promptly have significant benefit over and above those where there is delay in terms of morbidity and mortality [3].

However, the reality of daily practice is that many patients have blood pressure measured only infrequently and when they do have it measured it is done only once per session [4]. Therefore titration on the basis of clinic blood pressure measurements in primary care may be suboptimal. This has led to work considering the place of home/self-monitoring in guiding the titration of antihypertensive medication by health professionals [5–7]. Imai and colleagues' work showed that self-monitored blood pressure is highly reproducible [8]. Over and above this, interest in increased engagement with patient in controlling their own blood pressure has led to studies assessing self-management [9, 10]. This chapter reviews this evidence for the use of self-monitored blood pressure by both professionals and patients to titrate antihypertensive medication. The methods used for titration in each trial are outlined in Table 7.1.

7.2   Professional Led Titration of Antihypertensive Medication

Staessen et al.'s THOP trial published in JAMA in 2004 was the first to examine the efficacy of antihypertensive titration using self-monitored blood pressure [5]. Four hundred people with a diastolic blood pressure of 95 mmHg or more were randomised to antihypertensive medication titration either using home monitored diastolic blood pressure (average of six readings per day for a week) or carefully measured clinic diastolic blood pressure (mean of three sitting clinic readings). Medication was increased, reduced or left the same using a target range of diastolic blood pressure of 80–89 mmHg which was the same regardless of the setting of the blood pressure measurements. After an average of just under 12 months follow-up, blood pressure was significantly higher in the self-monitored group compared to the clinic monitored group: mean difference on 24 h ABPM (primary outcome) was 4.9/2.9 mmHg. More self-monitored BP patients had stopped medication: 25.6% vs. 11.3%; $P < 0.001$.

Similarly, the HOMERUS Trial compared antihypertensive medication titration using self-monitored or clinic monitored blood pressure with identical targets of 140/90 mmHg [6, 11]. Titration was again undertaken by a clinician blinded to randomisation group. After 1 year, ambulatory 24 h blood pressure was lower in those receiving treatment based on clinic measurement: 123.8/76.1 vs. 125.9/77.2 mmHg. Interestingly   office   measurements   were   very   similar: 142.2/84.3   vs. 143.8/85.4 mmHg. The self-monitoring group used less medication resulting in lower costs and importantly no difference was seen in either left ventricular mass of median urinary microalbumin concentration.

Both of these studies had important drawbacks when considering their relevance for physicians titrating antihypertensives [5, 11]: they used identical targets for home and clinic blood pressure whereas guidelines since have consistently recommended lower blood pressure targets for home measurements of 135/85 mmHg compared to a standard clinic target of 140/90 mmHg [12–14]. Both maintained blinding with a prescribing physician unaware of randomisation group; however,

Table 7.1 Trials using self-monitoring to titrate antihypertensives by physicians or patients

Author, year	HBPM basis for titration	Home target	Clinic BP measurement used for titration	Clinic target	Outcome
Staessen, 2004 THOP [5]	3 measurements after 5 min rest twice daily for 7 days. Mean of all readings in last 7 days	140/90: mmHg Blinded single investigator adjusting medication	Mean of 3 consecutive measurements made during usual clinic hours after 5 min rest	140/90: mmHg Blinded single investigator adjusting medication	24 h ABPM: mean difference between groups in favour of clinic monitoring: 4.9 mmHg (95% confidence intervals 2.5, 7.4)/2.9 (1.4, 4.4) 12 m
Verberk, 2007 HOMERUS [11]	BP measured for 7 days: three readings each in the morning and in the evening. Mean of 7 consecutive days of measurements	140/90: mmHg Blinded single investigator adjusting medication	Mean of blood pressure measured three times in sitting position after 5 min of rest with an interval of 2 min	140/90: mmHg Blinded single investigator adjusting medication	Clinic BP: mean difference (HBPM-CBPM) −1.6 (−5.3, 2.0)/−1.0 (−2.9, 0.9), i.e. no difference. For ABPM, mean difference (HBPM-CBPM): −2.1 (−4.3 to 0.0)/−1.1 (−2.7 to 0.4) mmHg 12 m
Stergiou, 2013 [15]	7 routine workdays within 2 weeks, with duplicate self-measurements in the morning (6–9 am, before drug intake if treated) and the evening (6–9 pm) after 5 min sitting rest and with 1 min between measurements	135/85 mmHg	Duplicate BP measurements were taken by a doctor after 5 min sitting rest and with a 1-min interval between measurements	140/90 mmHg	Mean difference in left ventricular mass index (HBPM-CBPM): 0.50 (−1.70, 2.70) g/m² 12 m
McKinstry, 2013 HITS [16]	Initial BP measured twice each morning and evening for a week and then weekly once BP controlled. Rolling average of last ten readings used in titration	135/85 mmHg	GP usual care: clinic readings measured using usual practice	140/90 mmHg	Mean difference in daytime systolic ambulatory blood pressure adjusted for baseline and minimisation factors (CBPM-HBPM): 4.3 mmHg (95% confidence interval 2.0 to 6.5; P = 0.0002) and for daytime diastolic ambulatory blood pressure was 2.3 mmHg (0.9 to 3.6; P = 0.001) 6 m

(continued)

Table 7.1 (continued)

Author, year	HBPM basis for titration	Home target	Clinic BP measurement used for titration	Clinic target	Outcome
McManus, 2018 TASMINH4 [7]	Blood pressure measured twice each morning and evening for 1 week per month. Mean of measurements on days 2–7 used for titration. Both telemonitoring and self-monitoring alone intervention groups	135/85 mmHg	GP usual care: clinic readings measured using usual practice	140/90 mmHg	Adjusted mean differences vs. usual care: self-monitoring alone, −3.5 mmHg [95% CI −5.8 to −1.2]; telemonitoring, −4.7 mmHg [−7.0 to −2.4]) 12 m
McManus, 2010 TASMINH2 [10]	Two readings each morning for 7 days; second reading used in calculation. Titration recommended if BP > 130/85 mmHg on 4 or more days in seven	130/85 mmHg	GP usual care: clinic readings measured using usual practice.	140/90 mmHg	Systolic blood pressure decreased by 17.6 mmHg (14.9–20.3) in the self-management group and by 12.2 mmHg (9.5–14.9) in the control group (difference between groups 5.4 mmHg, 2.4–8.5; $p = 0.0004$) 12 m
McManus, 2014 TASMINSR [9]	Two readings each morning for 7 days; second reading used in calculation. Titration recommended if BP > 120/80 mmHg on 4 or more days in seven	120/85 mmHg	GP usual care: clinic readings measured using usual practice	140/90 mmHg	Mean difference of 9.2 mmHg (95% CI, 5.7–12.7) in systolic and 3.4 mmHg (95% CI, 1.8–5.0) in diastolic blood pressure (CBPM-HBPM)

this meant that titration was arguably not similar to usual care. In THOP both groups received both types of measurement with ABPM as the outcome whereas in HOMERUS each group received ABPM but either home or clinic measurement. Finally, the titration was on the basis of diastolic blood pressure only in THOP and both systolic and diastolic in HOMERUS. Despite these differences, the results were similar showing less medication but higher blood pressure associated with the use of home monitoring, probably due to the fact that having an identical home and clinic target resulted in under treatment.

Stergiou et al. randomised 145 subjects (mean age 51, 60% male) with elevated but untreated blood pressure to management based on clinic and ABPM measurement or HBPM alone [15]. Their outcome was target organ damage assessed via echocardiographic left ventricular mass index (LVMI, primary endpoint), pulse wave velocity, and urinary albumin excretion. Identical stepped treatment strategies were used in both arms with HBPM used in one arm to check for BP control with a combination of clinic and ABPM measurements used in the other. Home and awake ABPM targets (135/85 mmHg for those at low/moderate risk) were lower than clinic targets (140/90 mmHg). After 1 year there was no significant difference between groups in LVMI or the secondary end points suggesting that the two strategies were equivalent.

McKinstry and colleagues in the HITS trial assessed a telemonitoring-based intervention with participants randomised to self-monitoring with a blue tooth connection to a telemonitoring site [16]. Self-monitoring was initially twice daily for a week and thereafter at least weekly. Clinicians had access to their patients' results through a web interface with indications of those above target backing up training around the same. Patients' BP measurements were automatically submitted via a Bluetooth link between their monitor and mobile phone and in addition they could opt into both online access to their blood pressure results and reports via text or email giving running averages of their blood pressure. Follow-up was again by ambulatory monitoring, this time after 6 months. The results showed a significant reduction in blood pressure in the self-monitoring group compared to control: mean difference in ABPM between groups 4.3/2.3 mmHg. This effect seemed to be mediated through increased prescription of antihypertensives to those that self-monitored and costs were £109 greater in the intervention group per person per 6 months, driven largely by the costs of the intervention (£71, (65% of the total cost)).

HITS involved a pragmatic intervention which was well accepted and showed clear benefits albeit with relatively short follow-up. The costs of the intervention were appreciable (not least because of increased use of professional consultation). Telemonitoring costs might be expected to drop over time. Nevertheless, with around 1:6 receiving treatment for hypertension in the UK alone, national implementation would likely need a cheaper system that did not impact on health care professional workload. Such a regime is being implemented in Scotland via the Scale-Up BP programme [17]. Because the feedback in HITS was optional it is hard to know what if any effect that might have had. Interestingly some professionals objected to feedback regarding patients just over target which on a population level can have significantly increased risk compared to those below target.

Most recently, the TASMINH4 study aimed to assess both the longer term (12 month) effect of titration using self-monitored blood pressure as well as to understand the influence of telemonitoring over and above self-monitoring with simple paper-based feedback [7]. 1182 hypertensive patients aged over 35 with blood pressure not controlled to below 140/90 mmHg were randomised to either hypertension management based on clinic readings or self-monitoring. Two separate groups utilising self-monitoring were studied: self-monitoring using paper charts to record blood pressure with monthly posting of results to the GP and self-monitoring with a simple text-based telemonitoring system. This incorporated automated feedback recommending professional consultation for both very high and low readings plus when averages went above target. Clinic targets were 140/90 mmHg whereas home targets were 135/85 mmHg as per international guidelines [12, 18].

After 12 months, both self-monitoring groups had significantly lower systolic blood pressure than those titrated against clinic readings with similar resource use: self-monitoring, 137·0 mmHg and telemonitoring, 136.0 mmHg vs. usual care, 140·4 mmHg. Prescription of antihypertensives was modestly increased in the self-monitoring groups. Economic modelling suggested that self-monitoring was likely to be cost-effective compared to usual care provided that the blood pressure reductions were maintained for at least 3 years following the trial, an assumption that seems acceptable based on similar work [19, 20].There was a fine balance between self-monitoring and telemonitoring both in terms of blood pressure and cost-effectiveness. Qualitative work suggested that telemonitoring reduced workload within practices by presenting averages and summaries of readings and that this would be further improved with integration into clinical record systems. However, both clinicians and patients felt that the option of self-monitoring alone should be available for individuals that found telemonitoring difficult.

The telemonitoring system used in the TASMINH4 trial used SMS messaging rather than "apps" due to issues with the market penetrance of smart phones at the time of the research. The algorithms underpinning the telemonitoring could be implemented within such apps and it seems likely that this, perhaps with the option of a Bluetooth connection, might be a route for implementation in the future, provided costs were not excessive.

Overall, these data suggest that physicians using self-monitoring to titrate antihypertensive medication can achieve better blood pressure control than when clinic monitoring is used. The key seems to be to implement the 135/85 mmHg target for home readings and to use self-monitoring on an ongoing basis. If a telemonitoring system is used it should be simple, with feedback to both professionals and patients. Patients should be given a choice as to whether they use telemonitoring.

7.3   Patient Self-Monitoring with Self-Titration

Even before the original work by Staessen et al. on professional titration using self-monitored blood pressure, the question arose whether patients could self-titrate using their own blood pressure readings to guide their own care. Other conditions such as diabetes and asthma had promoted such approaches for some time with success. Hypertension was perhaps different due to the largely asymptomatic nature of the condition but as management could be guided with accurate and easy to use electronic monitors then self-titration seemed possible.

Initial work came in the form of a small-scale trial in Canada where 31 hypertensive individuals were randomised 2:1 to a patient specific fixed self-titration schedule with follow-up over 2 months [21]. Those randomised to patient directed care had small but significant differences in blood pressure reduction compared to usual care but follow-up was after 8 weeks. Surprisingly, these promising early results were not taken forward until 10 years later when the TASMINH2 trial randomised 552 patients to self-monitoring with self-titration and followed them up for a year. Those in the intervention group used a primitive telemonitoring system and adjusted their medication following two predefined medication changes before needing to see their primary care physician for a further two changes. Those in the intervention group had 5.4/2.7 mmHg lower blood pressure after 1 year compared to control: 134.9/77.4 vs. 140.1/79.5 mmHg. This appeared to be mediated through increased use of medication in the self-managing group (around 0.5 additional antihypertensive medications per patient compared to control), with minimal difference in adverse effects. Those who self-managed made 55% of the changes recommended by their titration algorithms compared to around 45% in Bosworth's trial of physician titration [22].

The TASMIN-SR trial developed the concept of self-management, this time with patients able to make three medication changes agreed by primary care physicians at baseline based on the results of self-monitoring before needing to re-consult. The intervention was compared to usual care and this time the population comprised people with hypertension and at least one cardiometabolic co-morbidity (previous cardiovascular disease, diabetes, chronic kidney disease or any combination thereof). After 12 months, the mean blood pressure had decreased to 128.2/73.8 mm Hg in the intervention group and to 137.8/76.3 mm Hg in the control group, a difference of 9.2/3.4 mm Hg after correction for baseline blood pressure. Again, increased medication use in the intervention group seemed to be the mediator with just under one daily dose of antihypertensive medication increase in the self-management group. Interestingly, despite the older age (69 vs. 66 in TASMINH2) and higher cardiovascular risk, patients in this trial had better fidelity to the intervention with 70% of recommended medication changes being implemented [23].

7.4 Operational Concerns

The evidence for the efficacy of self-monitoring for the titration of antihypertensive medication is now robust but there are several operational issues that need to be considered in terms of implementation

(a) *International Guidelines:* the 2018 ESC/ESH guidelines for hypertension endorse much greater use of self-monitoring than previously and specifically in quantifying the effects of treatment, i.e. guiding antihypertensive medication titration. Clinicians can be confident that implementation of the evidence outlined in this chapter is in line with current recommendations.

(b) The use of *telemonitoring*: the data presented above suggests a significant place for telemonitoring in terms of ease of implementation but that it may not be appropriate for all individuals. The self-management work did not definitively provide evidence for telemonitoring in that context but ongoing work may clarify that situation.

(c) *Integration* of self-monitoring with clinical records: most trials to date have utilised bespoke systems to deliver BP measurement results to clinicians, typically using blue tooth or text-based systems linked to a web site. Ideally self-monitored blood pressure would be delivered directly to the clinical record in a manageable fashion; however, this potential has yet to be realised on a large scale.

(d) *How to choose patients* for self-titration: trials by necessity tend to include relatively small groups of motivated individuals but the true impact of an intervention will only be clear when it is offered more widely. It is not currently known how many patients adjust their own medication, with or without their physician's knowledge. A pragmatic solution would be to offer self-titration to all but to accept that take up may be by a relatively small proportion.

(e) *Reimbursement by insurance companies* in fee paying health care systems is often dependent on face-to-face consultations with telephone or remote consulting less financially recompensed or even not recompensed at all. The implementation of self-monitoring with or without self-titration as part of the cornerstone of hypertension care will require new ways of working and sensible reimbursement practices by relevant stakeholders.

7.5   Conclusions

This chapter has reviewed the evidence for antihypertensive titration using self-monitored blood pressure to guide changes both by clinicians and by their patients. A series of trials have been described, initially showing worse control using self-monitoring with equivalent targets to clinic monitoring but latterly better results from self-monitoring: provided standard (and lower, i.e. 135/85 mmHg) home targets are used, better blood pressure control is achieved through the use of self-monitoring, mediated through increased prescription of medication. Patients too can use self-monitored blood pressure to titrate their own antihypertensive medication successfully as shown in the TASMINH2 and TASMINSR studies. Because self-monitoring lowers blood pressure at little additional cost, cost-effectiveness analyses are generally positive. Self-monitoring should be a standard recommendation, with or without self-titration, for all patients with hypertension who are willing and able. Clinicians can feel confident that the use of self-monitoring should improve blood pressure control and do so in a cost-effective manner.

References

1. Effects of Treatment on Morbidity in Hypertension. Results in patients with diastolic blood pressures averaging 115 through 129 mmHg. JAMA. 1967;202(11):1028–34.
2. Hypertension Detection and Follow-Up Program Cooperative Group. Five-year findings of the hypertension detection and follow-up program. I. Reduction in mortality of persons with high blood pressure, including mild hypertension. JAMA. 1979;242(23):2562–71.
3. Xu W, Goldberg SI, Shubina M, Turchin A. Optimal systolic blood pressure target, time to intensification, and time to follow-up in treatment of hypertension: population based retrospective cohort study. BMJ. 2015;350:h158.
4. Stevens SL, McManus RJ, Stevens RJ. Current practice of usual clinic blood pressure measurement in people with and without diabetes: a survey and prospective 'mystery shopper' study in UK primary care. BMJ Open. 2018;8(4):e020589.
5. Staessen JA, Den Hond E, Celis H, Fagard R, Keary L, Vandenhoven G, et al. Antihypertensive treatment based on blood pressure measurement at home or in the physician's office: a randomized controlled trial. JAMA. 2004;291(8):955–64.
6. Verberk WJ, Kroon AA, Kessels AG, Dirksen C, Nelemans PJ, Lenders JW, et al. Home versus office blood pressure MEasurements: reduction of unnecessary treatment study: rationale and study design of the HOMERUS trial. Blood Press. 2003;12(5–6):326–33.
7. McManus RJ, Mant J, Franssen M, Nickless A, Schwartz C, Hodgkinson J, et al. Efficacy of self-monitored blood pressure, with or without telemonitoring, for titration of antihypertensive medication (TASMINH4): an unmasked randomised controlled trial. Lancet. 2018;391(10124):949–59.
8. Imai Y, Ohkubo T, Hozawa A, Tsuji I, Matsubara M, Araki T, et al. Usefulness of home blood pressure measurements in assessing the effect of treatment in a single-blind placebo-controlled open trial. J Hypertens. 2001;19(2):179–85.
9. McManus RJ, Mant J, Haque MS, Bray EP, Bryan S, Greenfield SM, et al. Effect of self-monitoring and medication self-titration on systolic blood pressure in hypertensive patients at high risk of cardiovascular disease: the TASMIN-SR randomized clinical trial. JAMA. 2014;312(8):799–808.
10. McManus RJ, Mant J, Bray EP, Holder R, Jones MI, Greenfield S, et al. Telemonitoring and self-management in the control of hypertension (TASMINH2): a randomised controlled trial. Lancet. 2010;376(9736):163–72.
11. Verberk WJ, Kroon AA, Lenders JW, Kessels AG, van Montfrans GA, Smit AJ, et al. Self-measurement of blood pressure at home reduces the need for antihypertensive drugs: a randomized, controlled trial. Hypertension. 2007;50(6):1019–25.
12. Krause T, Lovibond K, Caulfield M, McCormack T, Williams B. Management of hypertension: summary of NICE guidance. BMJ. 2011;343:d4891.
13. Whelton PK, Carey RM, Aronow WS, Casey DE Jr, Collins KJ, Dennison Himmelfarb C, et al. 2017 ACC/AHA/AAPA/ABC/ACPM/AGS/APhA/ASH/ASPC/NMA/PCNA guideline for the prevention, detection, evaluation, and management of high blood pressure in adults: a report of the American College of Cardiology American Heart Association task force on clinical practice guidelines. Hypertension. 2018;71(6):1269–24.
14. Williams B, Mancia G, Spiering W, Agabiti Rosei E, Azizi M, Burnier M, et al. 2018 ESC/ESH guidelines for the management of arterial hypertension: the task force for the management of arterial hypertension of the European Society of Cardiology and the European Society of Hypertension: the task force for the management of arterial hypertension of the European Society of Cardiology and the European Society of Hypertension. J Hypertens. 2018;36(10):1953–2041.
15. Stergiou GS, Karpettas N, Destounis A, Tzamouranis D, Nasothimiou E, Kollias A, et al. Home blood pressure monitoring alone vs. combined clinic and ambulatory measurements in following treatment-induced changes in blood pressure and organ damage. Am J Hypertens. 2014;27(2):184–92.

16. McKinstry B, Hanley J, Wild S, Pagliari C, Paterson M, Lewis S, et al. Telemonitoring based service redesign for the management of uncontrolled hypertension: multicentre randomised controlled trial. BMJ. 2013;346:f3030.
17. Scale-up blood pressure project: University of Edinburgh; 2018. https://www.ed.ac.uk/usher/telescot/projects/scale-up-bp.
18. Pickering TG, Miller NH, Ogedegbe G, Krakoff LR, Artinian NT, Goff D. Call to action on use and reimbursement for home blood pressure monitoring: a joint scientific statement from the American Heart Association, American Society Of Hypertension, and Preventive Cardiovascular Nurses Association. Hypertension. 2008;52(1):10–29.
19. Maciejewski ML, Bosworth HB, Olsen MK, Smith VA, Edelman D, Powers BJ, et al. Do the benefits of participation in a hypertension self-management trial persist after patients resume usual care? Circ Cardiovasc Qual Outcomes. 2014;7(2):269–75.
20. Monahan M, Jowett S, Nickless A, Franssen M, Grant S, Greenfield S, Hobbs FDR, Hodgkinson J, Mant J, McManus RJ. Cost-effectiveness of telemonitoring and self-monitoring of blood pressure for antihypertensive titration in primary care (TASMINH4). Hypertension. 2019;73(6):1231–9. https://doi.org/10.1161/HYPERTENSIONAHA.118.12415.
21. Zarnke KB, Feagan BG, Mahon JL, Feldman RD. A randomized study comparing a patient-directed hypertension management strategy with usual office-based care. Am J Hypertens. 1997;10(1):58–67.
22. Crowley MJ, Smith VA, Olsen MK, Danus S, Oddone EZ, Bosworth HB, et al. Treatment intensification in a hypertension telemanagement trial: clinical inertia or good clinical judgment? Hypertension. 2011;58(4):552–8.
23. Schwartz CL, Seyed-Safi A, Haque S, Bray EP, Greenfield S, Hobbs FDR, et al. Do patients actually do what we ask: patient fidelity and persistence to the targets and self-Management for the Control of blood pressure in stroke and at risk groups blood pressure self-management intervention. J Hypertens. 2018;36(8):1753–61.

Home Blood Pressure Monitoring, Treatment Adherence and Hypertension Control

8

Alejandro de la Sierra, Anastasia Mihailidou,
Ji-Guang Wang, Daichi Shimbo, and Richard J. McManus

Home blood pressure monitoring (HBPM) has been increasingly recognized as a useful tool for diagnosis and management of patients with suspected or confirmed BP elevation. Current guidelines [1, 2] now include HBPM due to its advantages in confirming hypertension, detection of white-coat and masked hypertension phenotypes, and its ability to improve monitoring of treated patients in order to make better decisions regarding such treatment.

In addition to these two main indications for HBPM, other additional advantages include the possibility of increasing treatment adherence and persistence by the use of HBPM, either as an isolated intervention or as part of a group of behavioural

A. de la Sierra (✉)
Department of Internal Medicine, Hospital Mutua Terrassa, University of Barcelona,
Barcelona, Catalonia, Spain
e-mail: adelasierra@mutuaterrassa.cat

A. Mihailidou
Cardiovascular & Hormonal Research Laboratory, Department of Cardiology and Kolling
Institute, Royal North Shore Hospital, Sydney, NSW, Australia

Macquarie University, Sydney, NSW, Australia
e-mail: anastasia.mihailidou@health.nsw.gov.au

J.-G. Wang
The Shanghai Institute of Hypertension, Ruijin Hospital, Shanghai Jiaotong University
School of Medicine, Shanghai, China

D. Shimbo
Department of Medicine, Columbia University Medical Center, New York, NY, USA
e-mail: ds2231@cumc.columbia.edu

R. J. McManus
Nuffield Department of Primary Care Health Sciences, University of Oxford,
Radcliffe Observatory Quarter, Oxford, UK
e-mail: richard.mcmanus@phc.ox.ac.uk

interventions, which may include telemonitoring and telemedicine. Moreover, the use of HBPM seems to be associated with an increased probability of achieving BP control, through different putative mechanisms, which again include an increase in the adherence to antihypertensive treatment, but also other lifestyle changes as a result of a deeper engagement with the patient leading to a better control of the disease.

We review here the available data regarding the use of HBPM and its impact on medication adherence and BP control.

8.1   HBPM and Medication Adherence

Medication adherence can be defined as the process by which patients take their medication as prescribed. Adherence is a dynamic process which includes treatment initiation, execution (correct implementation of the dose regimen) and persistence [3]. Low adherence is the most common cause of treatment resistance [4] and it is associated with an increased risk of cardiovascular events [5]. Strategies focused on improving adherence are complex and related to patient's behaviour and education, physician attitude, complexity of drug regimen and other health care supportive measures [3].

HBPM has been proposed as one of the strategies which may improve adherence. To date, several studies, one systematic review and one meta-analysis have reported data on the effect of HBPM in adherence improvement. In 2006, Ogedegbe and Schoenthaler [6] reviewed eleven randomized controlled trials, from which six reported improvements in medication adherence. However, in most of these trials HBPM was used in combination with other interventions, such as patient counselling, additional education, or medication reminders, thus resulting in difficulties in establishing the specific role of each component.

In one of the studies of HBPM as an isolated intervention, the authors reported a significant increase in the number of pills taken per week, from 5.8 to 6.6, assessed by electronic monitoring after 6 weeks of intervention in 628 patients [7]. In a second study, with a considerable smaller sample (60 patients), HBPM produced a non-significant ($p > 0.05$) increase in adherence (94% versus 88%) [8].

A total of 28 trials with more than 7000 participants were included in a meta-analysis of the effect of HBPM on medication adherence [9]. Again, most studies [10] combined HBPM with other co-interventions, with only 11 examining the role of HBPM alone. Adherence was assessed by different methods, including electronic monitoring, pill count, pharmacy fill data, and self-report adherence. A pooled analysis of 13 studies with quantitative data revealed a significant modest effect of HBPM (isolated or associated to other co-interventions) in medication adherence with a standardized mean difference of 0.21 (95% CI: 0.08–0.34).

These results are not easy to interpret, as two important confounders may either enhance or reduce the importance of HBPM in the adherence issue. First, as aforementioned, most of the studies included a mixture of interventions, with HBPM being only a part of them. The positive results derived from these studies could be either an effect of HBPM, of other interventions or a mixture of them. Another important aspect to be taken into account is how representative was the sample included in studies of adherence of the general population with hypertension. It is well known that most participants in such studies are highly motivated often exhibiting high levels of adherence at baseline, not necessarily representing the actual level of medication adherence in the general population with hypertension where 25% will never even fill a prescription for a new medication. High levels of adherence at baseline obviously reduce the possibility of any intervention impacting on such adherence.

8.2   HBPM and BP Control

The use of HBPM is associated with improved BP control compared to conventional management based on office BP measurements [11–14]. Several meta-analyses have reported small although significant reduction in both systolic and diastolic BP in patients using HBPM. In 2001, Cappuccio et al. [11] reviewed 18 randomized controlled trials and found a reduction of 4.2/2.4 mmHg with HBPM, these differences remaining significant (2.2/1.9 mmHg) after adjusting for publication bias. Several years later Agarwal et al. [12] reviewed 37 randomized controlled trials and also found significant reductions (2.6/1.7 mmHg) in BP. Additional findings were that BP reduction were more pronounced when HBPM was complemented with telemonitoring. Furthermore, HBPM led to more frequent down-titrations in antihypertensive therapy and was associated with less therapeutic inertia.

Two more recent meta-analyses have also found small, although significant, effects of HBPM on BP values. Uhlig et al. [13], in a meta-analysis of 26 comparative studies, found a significant effect of HBPM at 6 months (3.9/2.4 mmHg). The results were considered of moderate-strength evidence. However, changes after 1 year (1.5/0.8 mmHg) were no longer significant. In studies combining HBPM with other co-interventions, the beneficial effect on BP remained significant after 1 year. Finally, Tucker et al. [14] reported another meta-analysis which was based on individual patient data from 25 trials which included more than 7000 patients. Results revealed a lack of significant effect of HBPM alone, although its combination with other supportive co-interventions was associated with lower BP at 12 months.

As with medication adherence, the impact of HBPM on BP values appears heterogeneous, depending on the presence of other lifestyle changes, the method of treatment modification and also the use of different or the same targets for clinic or home BP.

8.3   HBPM in the Context of Self-Management

A constant finding in studies assessing the effect of HBPM on either adherence or BP control is that such intervention seems to be more efficacious when is accompanied by other co-interventions. Among them, self-management and telemonitoring have been studied more in depth.

The TASMINH2 study [15] examined the effect of self-management, consisting of self-titration of antihypertensive medication, in comparison with usual care in patients with uncomplicated hypertension whose systolic BP was not controlled while on two or less antihypertensive medications. Telemonitoring was also included in the intervention group, for safety purposes. The primary outcome (reduction in systolic BP) was significant in favour of the intervention group (mean difference 3.7 mmHg and 5.4 mmHg at 6 and 12 months, respectively).

These results were also reproduced in high-risk individuals with hypertension, defined by systolic BP above 130/80 mmHg and a history of stroke, coronary heart disease, diabetes or chronic kidney disease [16]. Corresponding differences in systolic and diastolic BP at 12 months were 9.2 and 3.4 mmHg, respectively.

The main limitation of studies reporting benefits of self-management is the generalizability to the whole population with hypertension, as not all patients are suitable for engagement in such self-management.

8.4 HBPM in the Context of Telemonitoring

Telemonitoring can be an alternative to self-management. The use of automated devices that are able to transmit the data to health care providers (usually physicians, nurses or pharmacists) has allowed the study of the effect of remote management on BP control. A clinical trial in US individuals with hypertension reported 12-month reductions of 11/6 mmHg for systolic and diastolic BP, in patients using transmission of data and receiving treatment adjustments from their pharmacist, when compared to usual care [17]. An extended analysis of the same cohort suggested that the effect remained clinically significant 1 year after the intervention was stopped, but was negligible 4 years later [10].

Meta-analyses focused on the antihypertensive effect of intervention based on HBP telemonitoring have revealed a significant effect on BP control (16% increase in the possibility of achieving such control) with an effect on BP reduction of 4–5 mmHg for systolic and 2–3 mmHg for diastolic BP [18, 19]. These results were accompanied by an increase in antihypertensive medication use without differences in adherence, number of office consultations or changes in the quality of life.

A recent trial has examined the effect of telemonitoring added to self-measurement alone on BP reduction. The TASMINH4 study [20] enrolled 1182 patients with hypertension from the UK, randomized to usual care (therapeutic decisions based on clinic BP measurements), self-monitoring alone (therapeutic decisions based on HBPM, with readings sent to the physicians one per month) and telemonitoring (data transmitted through SMS). In both intervention groups, physicians were asked to review the data once per month and to adjust antihypertensive treatment based on HBPM readings. After 12 months, both intervention groups had lower systolic BP in comparison to usual care (3.5 mmHg for self-monitoring alone and 4.7 mmHg for telemonitoring) without significant differences between them. Moreover, as observed in previous TASMIN studies [15, 16], patients engaged in self-monitoring had an increased medication use [20].

These results confirm that HBPM is a useful tool for achieving a better BP control, if used on a scheduled basis and when adjustments in antihypertensive treatment are based on such readings. Telemonitoring did not seem to add advantages in such experimental context, although it could be obviously useful in other circumstances, such as difficulties in access to physicians or in cases of doubts regarding the reliability of the data.

In conclusion, most of the trials suggest that the impact of HBPM on BP control and treatment adherences is more powerful if used in a context of other interventions, such as lifestyles changes, as well as other interventions that are able to improve adherence and to increase the implication of the patient in his/her management.

References

1. Whelton PK, Carey RM, Aronow WS, Casey DE Jr, Collins KJ, Dennison Himmelfarb C, et al. 2017 ACC/AHA/AAPA/ABC/ACPM/AGS/APhA/ASH/ASPC/NMA/PCNA guideline for the prevention, detection, evaluation, and management of high blood pressure in adults: executive summary: a report of the American College of Cardiology/American Heart Association task force on clinical practice guidelines. Hypertension. 2018;71(6):1269–324.
2. Williams B, Mancia G, Spiering W, Agabiti Rosei E, Azizi M, Burnier M, et al. 2018 ESC/ESH guidelines for the management of arterial hypertension: the task force for the management of arterial hypertension of the European Society of Cardiology and the European Society of Hypertension: the task force for the management of arterial hypertension of the European Society of Cardiology and the European Society of Hypertension. J Hypertens. 2018;36(10):1953–2041.
3. Vrijens B, Antoniou S, Burnier M, de la Sierra A, Volpe M. Current situation of medication adherence in hypertension. Front Pharmacol. 2017;8:100.
4. Jung O, Gechter JL, Wunder C, Paulke A, Bartel C, Geiger H, et al. Resistant hypertension? Assessment of adherence by toxicological urine analysis. J Hypertens. 2013;31(4):766–74.
5. Corrao G, Parodi A, Nicotra F, Zambon A, Merlino L, Cesana G, et al. Better compliance to antihypertensive medications reduces cardiovascular risk. J Hypertens. 2011;29(3):610–8.
6. Ogedegbe G, Schoenthaler A. A systematic review of the effects of home blood pressure monitoring on medication adherence. J Clin Hypertens (Greenwich). 2006;8(3):174–80.
7. Vrijens B, Goetghebeur E. Comparing compliance patterns between randomized treatments. Control Clin Trials. 1997;18(3):187–203.
8. Bailey B, Carney SL, Gillies AA, Smith AJ. Antihypertensive drug treatment: a comparison of usual care with self blood pressure measurement. J Hum Hypertens. 1999;13(2):147–50.
9. Fletcher BR, Hartmann-Boyce J, Hinton L, McManus RJ. The effect of self-monitoring of blood pressure on medication adherence and lifestyle factors: a systematic review and meta-analysis. Am J Hypertens. 2015;28(10):1209–21.
10. Margolis KL, Asche SE, Dehmer SP, Bergdall AR, Green BB, Sperl-Hillen JM, et al. Long-term outcomes of the effects home blood pressure telemonitoring and pharmacist management on blood pressure among adults with uncontrolled hypertension. Follow-up of a cluster randomized clinical trial. JAMA Netw Open. 2018;1(5):e181617.
11. Cappuccio FP, Kerry SM, Forbes L, Donald A. Blood pressure control by home monitoring: meta-analysis of randomised trials. BMJ. 2004;329(7458):145.
12. Agarwal R, Bills JE, Hecht TJ, Light RP. Role of home blood pressure monitoring in overcoming therapeutic inertia and improving hypertension control: a systematic review and meta-analysis. Hypertension. 2011;57(1):29–38.

13. Uhlig K, Patel K, Ip S, Kitsios GD, Balk EM. Self-measured blood pressure monitoring in the management of hypertension: a systematic review and meta-analysis. Ann Intern Med. 2013;159(3):185–94.
14. Tucker KL, Sheppard JP, Stevens R, Bosworth HB, Bove A, Bray EP, et al. Self-monitoring of blood pressure in hypertension: a systematic review and individual patient data meta-analysis. PLoS Med. 2017;14(9):e1002389.
15. McManus RJ, Mant J, Bray EP, Holder R, Jones MI, Greenfield S, et al. Telemonitoring and self-management in the control of hypertension (TASMINH2): a randomised controlled trial. Lancet. 2010;376(9736):163–72.
16. McManus RJ, Mant J, Haque MS, Bray EP, Bryan S, Greenfield SM, et al. Effect of self-monitoring and medication self-titration on systolic blood pressure in hypertensive patients at high risk of cardiovascular disease: the TASMIN-SR randomized clinical trial. JAMA. 2014;312(8):799–808.
17. Margolis KL, Asche SE, Bergdall AR, Dehmer SP, Groen SE, Kadrmas HM, et al. Effect of home blood pressure telemonitoring and pharmacist management on blood pressure control: a cluster randomized clinical trial. JAMA. 2013;310(1):46–56.
18. Omboni S, Gazzola T, Carabelli G, Parati G. Clinical usefulness and cost effectiveness of home blood pressure telemonitoring: meta-analysis of randomized controlled studies. J Hypertens. 2013;31(3):455–67.
19. Duan Y, Xie Z, Dong F, Wu Z, Lin Z, Sun N, et al. Effectiveness of home blood pressure telemonitoring: a systematic review and meta-analysis of randomised controlled studies. J Hum Hypertens. 2017;31(7):427–37.
20. McManus RJ, Mant J, Franssen M, Nickless A, Schwartz C, Hodgkinson J, et al. Efficacy of self-monitored blood pressure, with or without telemonitoring, for titration of antihypertensive medication (TASMINH4): an unmasked randomised controlled trial. Lancet. 2018;391(10124):949–59.

Home Blood Pressure Monitoring: Cost-Effectiveness, Patients' Preference and Barriers for Clinical Use

9

Paul Muntner, Richard J. McManus, Daichi Shimbo, Alejandro de la Sierra, and Martin G. Myers

9.1   Introduction

Blood pressure (BP) is one of the most common measurements performed in clinical practice. Many guidelines from around the world recommend recording BP outside of the clinic setting to confirm a diagnosis of possible hypertension, prior to initiating antihypertensive medication [1–4]. Also, obtaining out-of-office BP readings is recommended for monitoring the control of blood pressure for patients taking antihypertensive medication. The most commonly used methods for measuring BP outside of the clinic setting are ambulatory blood pressure monitoring (ABPM)

P. Muntner (✉)
Department of Epidemiology, University of Alabama at Birmingham, Birmingham, AL, USA
e-mail: pmuntner@uab.edu

R. J. McManus
Nuffield Department of Primary Care Health Sciences, University of Oxford,
Radcliffe Observatory Quarter, Oxford, UK
e-mail: richard.mcmanus@phc.ox.ac.uk

D. Shimbo
Department of Medicine, Columbia University Medical Center, New York, NY, USA
e-mail: ds2231@cumc.columbia.edu

A. de la Sierra
Department of Internal Medicine, Hospital Mutua Terrassa, University of Barcelona,
Barcelona, Catalonia, Spain
e-mail: adelasierra@mutuaterrassa.cat

M. G. Myers
Division of Cardiology, Schulich Heart Program, Sunnybrook Health Sciences Centre,
Toronto, ON, Canada

Department of Medicine, University of Toronto, Toronto, ON, Canada
e-mail: martin.myers@sunnybrook.ca

© The Editor(s), under exclusive license to Springer Nature Switzerland AG 2020
G. S. Stergiou et al. (eds.), *Home Blood Pressure Monitoring*,
Updates in Hypertension and Cardiovascular Protection,
https://doi.org/10.1007/978-3-030-23065-4_9

and home blood pressure monitoring (HBPM) [5]. While many guidelines and scientific statements consider ABPM to be the reference standard for measuring BP, HBPM is often considered to be a reasonable alternative [6].

The decision to use ABPM or HBPM often reflects the preferences of the individual patient and those of the healthcare provider. The health system in which a patient receives care may also be a factor. Shared decision-making may play a large role in which technique is used for out-of-office BP monitoring, as both ABPM and HBPM appear reliable. It remains unclear whether one approach is superior to the other for diagnosing hypertension and monitoring control of BP. Clinicians can often guide the decision to use ABPM or HBPM based on which devices they have available and their preference. However, the use of ABPM or HBPM may be based ultimately on the patients' own viewpoint.

Hypertension is a lifelong condition and patients must be willing to monitor their BP outside of the office setting for ABPM or HBPM to be effective. Although HBPM involves patients in their own BP care, it also relies on the provider and other factors related to the healthcare system. Clinicians and healthcare systems can either facilitate access to HBPM or present barriers to its use. An appreciation of the barriers and facilitators to out-of-office testing as perceived by patients may facilitate clinicians' ability to provide patient-centered care. In this chapter, we review studies on patient and provider preferences for HBPM and the cost-effectiveness of HBPM.

9.2 Patient Preference

9.2.1 Results from Focus Groups

A number of researchers have conducted focus group discussions with patients to investigate their acceptance of HBPM. In a study conducted in the Netherlands, patients who had completed out-of-clinic BP monitoring with ABPM were recruited by their general practitioner and through social media [7]. None of the patients enrolled in this study had prior experience with HBPM. Patients reported HBPM would be useful, easier and more effective than ABPM since it would not interrupt their daily activity or cause pain/bruising.

In a separate set of focus groups conducted among patients who did not have hypertension and were recruited from clinics for low income populations in New York City, facilitators explained the concept of white coat hypertension and recommendations for ABPM and HBPM [8]. Many patients reported concerns about performing HBPM, including skepticism of the validity and reliability of devices, the challenges of arranging their schedule to obtain readings in the morning and evening and lack of confidence in performing the procedure. Also, the cost of buying a HBPM device was a concern for this low-income population. Patients reported a higher likelihood of performing HBPM if they were provided instructions on to how to conduct the procedure. HBPM was preferred over ABPM by some patients, as they perceived it to be more convenient and it would not disrupt their sleep. However, advantages of ABPM noted by patients included insurance coverage for the procedure, the involvement of medical staff setting up and initiating the device for testing, the limited time requirement (i.e., only 24 hours), and concerns about forgetfulness with HBPM.

A third set of focus groups was conducted in the United Kingdom and aimed at identifying the HBPM schedules that could increase its use and adherence [9]. These groups included patients who had participated in a trial of self-management of BP. Patients reported that having formal schedules could improve adherence to HBPM. It was recognized that obtaining more readings provided a more accurate estimate of BP, but that anxiety could also be experienced. Flexibility was deemed to be important with the HBPM schedule. Patients preferred a shorter schedule (e.g., 3 days) but stated they would comply with a 7 day schedule if was recommended by their healthcare provider.

9.2.2 Results from Structured Patient Surveys

Several studies have enrolled participants who have undergone both HBPM and ABPM and then asked about their preferred BP measurement approach. In 2002, Little and colleagues published data from 200 patients with newly diagnosed hypertension or with established hypertension and uncontrolled BP [10]. All participants had BP measured by a nurse, a doctor, in their own home (i.e., HBPM), and by ABPM. Patients reported HBPM to be associated with less anxiety than when BP was measured by a nurse or physician. It was also preferred due to the ability to avoid waiting around when compared to nurse or physician measured BP. Also, HBPM resulted in fewer disturbances and was more comfortable than ABPM. Finally, patients reported a greater feeling of self-control with HBPM and that it was a good way to save doctors' or nurses' time.

In 2007, Logan and colleagues published data from a survey of 142 patients with hypertension from the province of Ontario, Canada [11]. Overall, 78% of participants reported owning an HBPM device and 68% of participants had measured their BP at home in the past year. Most participants reported their own interest in BP was the most important reason for using HBPM. For participants who did not use HBPM, they reported it was because their doctor didn't tell them to (53%) and they preferred to have their BP measured by their doctor or medical staff (50%). Only 16% of participants reported not being confident enough to measure their BP at home and only 9% did not use HBPM because it made them more anxious.

In a study of 83 patients recruited from the Edinburgh, Scotland ABPM service who had undergone ABPM and HBPM, 81% preferred HBPM to ABPM [12]. The main reasons reported were the ability to instantly see their BP level, being more in control of obtaining BP measurements, less embarrassment in public, and HBPM did not interfere with their sleep. Only 16% of study participants reported having difficulty adhering to the time constraints required of HBPM and only 4% reported an increase in anxiety with HBPM. The 19% of patients who preferred ABPM over HBPM stated that it was because the procedure was over in 24 h. Additionally, the authors noted that the time required to explain the procedure to

Table 9.1 Patient preferences and concerns for conducting home blood pressure monitoring

Preferences	Concerns
• Does not interrupt daily activity • Does not cause pain/bruising • More convenient than ambulatory blood pressure monitoring • Does not disrupt sleep • Less anxiety than clinic-measured blood pressure • More self-control • Can save doctor/nurse time • Easy to perform	• Skepticism about device validity • Lack of confidence in performing home blood pressure monitoring • Cost of devices • Requires long-term commitment

patients was less for HBPM compared with ABPM (10–15 min for HBPM versus 30 min for ABPM).

In 2014, Nasothimiou and colleagues reported on a study wherein patients (n = 104) were randomized to undergo ABPM followed by HBPM or HBPM followed by ABPM [13]. After completing each test, a higher proportion of participants reported a positive opinion for HBPM (82%) versus ABPM (63%). Participants were more likely to request HBPM (60%) than ABPM (40%) if they needed to perform out-of-office BP monitoring again. HBPM was reported to be easy to perform by 95% of participants compared to only 61% for ABPM. Moderate to severe discomfort was reported for ABPM by 55% of participants versus only 13% for HBPM. Moderate/severe restriction of daily activity was reported for 30% of participants after undergoing ABPM versus 7% after HBPM.

Patient preferences and concerns for conducting HBPM are summarized in Table 9.1.

9.3   Healthcare Provider's Perspective

9.3.1   Focus Groups

In a series of nine nominal groups, 63 providers were asked to discuss and rank barriers and facilitators to conducting HBPM and ABPM [14]. Providers suggested that there were several barriers that prevented the use of HBPM in their clinic. These were grouped into themes according to the Theoretical Domains Framework. The most commonly reported barrier that prevented the conduct of HBPM related to beliefs about capability and consequences (e.g., ability of patients to correctly perform HBPM, test results being inaccurate due to the use of an invalid device or patients not following the BP measurement protocol). Additionally, the cost of the HBPM devices, low reimbursement to physicians, and lack of time to train patients were noted as barriers to performing HBPM. A second study that used focus group discussions with physicians in the Netherlands had similar findings. Specifically, physicians reported that HBPM was inferior to ABPM and that not all of their patients would be capable of conducting HBPM [7]. In this study, it was found that physicians discouraged the use of HBPM as they believed ABPM was a superior approach to measuring BP outside of the clinic setting.

9.3.2 Results from Structured Provider Surveys

In a study from a single health system in the US, more than 75% of providers completing a structured questionnaire on HBPM considered the procedure part of standard care in their practice [15]. Over 90% of providers who reported using HBPM said it was to guide treatment and two-thirds used it to improve adherence. Barriers to conducting HBPM included the lack of knowledge regarding validated devices and lack of data on the scientific evidence that HBPM will result in better BP control. Additionally, providers reported that patients' poor eyesight and lack of confidence would result in not obtaining valid BP measurements on HBPM. Also, a high proportion of providers (~40% to 50%) reported that they preferred measuring BP in the office setting. Nearly 33% thought that patients would be anxious if their BP was not controlled when measured on HBPM and over 40% of providers reported no one was available in their practice to teach patients how to properly conduct HBPM.

Among a random sample of all primary care providers in Hungary ($n = 405$; 58% response rate), 98.5% agreed that HBPM was part of standard of care and 94.4% often and almost always encouraged their patients to perform HBPM [16]. HBPM was considered to be equal or more important that office-based BP measurements by over 95% of providers. Despite the high proportion of providers who reported using HBPM, only 67% stated their service taught patients how to conduct HBPM. Barriers to conducting HBPM included concerns about the availability of validated devices (79%), that patients would become preoccupied with their BP (54%), and that most patients were not properly trained (40%). Also, over 25% of providers were concerned that the HBPM results would make their patients anxious and would result in frequent phone calls to the office. Facilitators to increase the use of HBPM included the availability of training facilities, inclusion of diagnostic and treatment protocols based on HBPM, programs that tabulate/display the HBPM results and evidence that it improved BP control.

In a third study, a random sample of primary care providers in Ontario, Canada, was mailed a survey on HBPM [11]. Among 478 providers (response rate 55%) who reported treating patients with hypertension, 52% considered HBPM part of standard of care and 63% often or almost always encouraged HBPM. Overall, 98% of providers reported using HBPM to detect white coat hypertension, 93% to guide antihypertensive treatment, 69% to improve medication adherence, and 56% to confirm the presence of resistant hypertension. Similar to the study in Hungary, a high percentage of providers reported barriers to HBPM with 70% being concerned that patients would become preoccupied with their BP and 65% uncertain of the accuracy of home devices. Also, 63% stated they would use HBPM more often if they had a list of validated devices, 49% if devices were more affordable and 45% if more evidence were available showing that HBPM improves BP. Only 5% of providers reported having someone in the office available to train patients.

Table 9.2 Healthcare provider concerns for conducting home blood pressure monitoring

Concerns
• Ability of patients to correctly perform home blood pressure monitoring
• Test results being inaccurate due to the use of an invalid device
• Patients not following the blood pressure measurement protocol
• Cost of the device
• Low reimbursement
• Lack of time to train patients
• Poor patient eyesight
• Patients' lack of confidence
• Patients would become anxious
• Lack of device availability

Finally, a structured telephone survey was conducted among primary care providers in Greece ($n = 366$; 87.4% participation rate) to investigate the implementation of HBPM guidelines [17]. Overall, 94% of providers reported using HBPM for their patients with hypertension. The most common indications were white coat hypertension, treatment titration, and detection of hypertension, while only 1% reported using HBPM to detect masked hypertension. Only 30% of providers based treatment decisions on the results of the HBPM. The main limitations noted for HBPM included 80% of providers who expressed concerns that patients were not reliable in reporting their BP and 41% who questioned the accuracy of the HBPM devices. Additionally, 86% of the providers who reported not using HBPM stated that they did not trust BP readings recorded by patients. While many patients do not accurately report their BP values on HBPM, this problem can be minimized by having patients use a device that stores readings and having them bring their device into the clinic [18]. Also, some HBPM devices have the capability of transmitting BP readings to the clinic which eliminates the need to rely on the accuracy of patients reporting their own BP [19].

Healthcare provider concerns with conducting HBPM are summarized in Table 9.2.

9.4   Cost-Effectiveness

The widespread implementation of HBPM may require data on its cost-effectiveness for diagnosing hypertension and managing BP among those with established hypertension. Data on the cost-effectiveness of HBPM have been generated from analyses of randomized controlled trials and simulation studies. Without other co-interventions, HBPM has been found to provide only a small BP lowering benefit that is not sustained over time [20, 21]. The BP-lowering benefit of HBPM has been greater when used with co-interventions (e.g., telemonitoring, pharmacist visits) [20]. Therefore, the cost-effectiveness of HBPM needs to be considered within the context of, and costs associated with, these co-interventions. When interpreting these data it is important to distinguish HBPM from the broader category of self-measured BP, which may also include the use of kiosks or measurements obtained by a patient using an automated device at their healthcare provider's office [22]. The section below focuses on HBPM and does not include studies that have investigated the cost-effectiveness of self-measurement protocols unless it was explicitly stated that HBPM was performed.

9.4.1 Data from Randomized Controlled Trials

A randomized trial conducted in the Kaiser Permanente Medical System evaluated the cost of HBPM versus usual care among 430 patients who were randomized at a 1:1 ratio to a HBPM intervention or usual care [23]. The intervention included receipt of a HBPM device with the request to measure BP twice weekly and mail a record of the recordings along with changes in medications/side effects every 4 weeks. After a 1-year intervention period, the decline in SBP and DBP were 3.3 mm Hg and 1.6 mm Hg larger among participants randomized to the HBPM intervention compared with usual care. Participants randomized to the HBPM intervention had 1.2 fewer office visits and 0.8 more telephone calls with medical staff compared to their counterparts randomized to usual care. In 1986 US dollars, the cost of hypertension care was lower in the HBPM versus usual care randomization arm ($88.28 versus $125.37). Even considering the cost of the HBPM device and patient training, the authors of this study concluded HBPM to be cost saving.

The cost-effectiveness of HBPM was evaluated in a randomized trial that showed HBPM in conjunction with clinical pharmacist specialist meetings reduced SBP by 21 mm Hg versus 8 mm Hg for those randomized to usual care [24]. Over 6 months of follow-up, the HBPM intervention was associated with hypertension-related costs of $455 per-patient versus $179 per-patient for those randomized to usual care. The higher costs with HBPM resulted from increased contact with healthcare providers, laboratory monitoring, medication use, and the HBPM device. HBPM did not reduce the need for outpatient, hospital or emergency department visits. Total healthcare costs were also higher among participants randomized to the intervention versus usual care ($1530 versus $1283). Extrapolating the BP-lowering of the HBPM intervention across the lifespan, it was associated with a favorable incremental cost-effectiveness ratio (ICER); $20.50 for each 1 mm Hg lowering of SBP and $3330 per additional life-year gained.

9.4.2 Modeling Studies

Using a Markov model based on healthcare expenditures in Japan and the prevalence of white coat hypertension from the Ohasama study, HBPM was reported to be associated with cost savings for the Japanese population (medical costs: $9.33 million US dollars [1.09 billion Yen] per 1000 patients over a five-year period with implementation of HBPM versus $10.89 US dollars [1.27 billion Yen] without implementation of HBPM) [25]. The authors reported that the cost-effectiveness of HBPM would be more favorable when conducted in populations with a higher prevalence of white coat hypertension and a lower annual transition rate from white coat hypertension to hypertension based on HBPM.

In a US-based study of patients with health insurance, a decision-analytic model was used to evaluate the short- and long-term cost-benefit and return on investment comparing HBPM versus BP recorded in the clinic setting for the diagnosis and treatment of hypertension [26]. From the health insurer's perspective, HBPM was associated with net savings that were higher at older age and increased over progressively longer follow-up. For example, over a 10-year time horizon, HBPM was estimated to result in cost-savings of $414.81, $439.14, and $1364.27 among adults 20–44, 45–64, and $\geq$ 65 years of age, respectively. When the cost-effectiveness of HBPM was divided into its use for the diagnosis versus treatment of hypertension, it was estimated that HBPM provided a better return on investment for diagnosis at younger ages and for guiding treatment at older ages.

Lovibond and colleagues conducted a Markov model-based analysis to compare the cost-effectiveness and quality adjusted life years gained when diagnosing hypertension based on BP recorded monthly in the clinic setting over 3 months and by HBPM over 1 week [27]. At each age evaluated (40, 50, 60, 70, and 75 years), diagnosing hypertension by HBPM and clinic-measured BP were equivalent in terms of costs and quality-adjusted life years gained for both men and women. However, HBPM was deemed to be cost-effective in sensitivity analyses wherein it was presumed to have the same sensitivity and specificity for identifying hypertension as ABPM or in younger age groups when the frequency of repeat monitoring following a normal results was reduced from 5 years to 1 year. A subsequent modeling analysis using data from the US reported HBPM to be associated with higher costs and lower quality-adjusted life years than using clinic-measured BP for the initial diagnosis of hypertension [28]. It should be noted that these studies were strongly influenced by the sensitivity and specificity of HBPM for diagnosing hypertension and there are few data available for generating these estimates [29]. Additionally, data are needed on the cost-effectiveness of screening for masked hypertension.

9.5   Conclusion

The value of HBPM for diagnosing hypertension and monitoring BP among individuals taking antihypertensive medication is well recognized. Data from several countries suggest that HBPM is preferred over ABPM by a majority of patients. While providers have concerns about their patients' ability to perform HBPM and the accuracy of devices used, they see potential benefits for their patients who conduct HBPM. There appear to be some discrepancies in the perception of HBPM between patients and providers. For example, providers believe that many patients will become anxious with the results of HBPM whereas patients do not report this concern. Published data on the cost-effectiveness of HBPM have been conflicting. Some analyses have suggested that HBPM may not be cost-effective for diagnosing hypertension. However, the results of these studies may have been heavily influenced by assumptions about the sensitivity and specificity of different approaches for identifying hypertension, an area for which few data are available. Additionally, data are needed on the cost-effectiveness of conducting HBPM for patients with suspected white coat hypertension and masked hypertension as recommended in clinical practice guidelines. Taken together, the preferences of patients and providers, and the cost-effectiveness data support the use of HBPM.

References

1. Whelton PK, Carey RM, Aronow WS, Casey DE Jr, Collins KJ, Dennison Himmelfarb C, et al. 2017 ACC/AHA/AAPA/ABC/ACPM/AGS/APhA/ASH/ASPC/NMA/PCNA guideline for the prevention, detection, evaluation, and Management of High Blood Pressure in adults: executive summary: a report of the American College of Cardiology/American Heart Association task Force on clinical practice guidelines. J Am Coll Cardiol. 2018;71:2199–269.
2. Leung AA, Daskalopoulou SS, Dasgupta K, McBrien K, Butalia S, Zarnke KB, et al. Hypertension Canada's 2017 guidelines for diagnosis, risk assessment, prevention, and treatment of hypertension in adults. Can J Cardiol. 2017;33:557–76.
3. Gabb GM, Mangoni AA, Anderson CS, Cowley D, Dowden JS, Golledge J, et al. Guideline for the diagnosis and management of hypertension in adults - 2016. Med J Aust. 2016;205:85–9.
4. Williams B, Mancia G, Agabiti Rosei E, Azizi M, Burnier M, Spiering W, et al. 2018 ESC/ESH guidelines for the management of arterial hypertension. Eur Heart J. 2018;39:3021–104.
5. Shimbo D, Abdalla M, Falzon L, Townsend RR, Muntner P. Role of ambulatory and home blood pressure monitoring in clinical practice: a narrative review. Ann Intern Med. 2015;163:691–700.
6. Siu AL, Force USPST. Screening for high blood pressure in adults: U.S. preventive services task Force recommendation statement. Ann Intern Med. 2015;163:778–86.
7. Carrera PM, Lambooij MS. Implementation of out-of-office blood pressure monitoring in the Netherlands: from clinical guidelines to Patients' adoption of innovation. Medicine (Baltimore). 2015;94:e1813.
8. Carter EJ, Moise N, Alcantara C, Sullivan AM, Kronish IM. Patient barriers and facilitators to ambulatory and home blood pressure monitoring: a qualitative study. Am J Hypertens. 2018;31:919–27.
9. Grant S, Hodgkinson JA, Milner SL, Martin U, Tompson A, Hobbs FR, et al. Patients' and clinicians' views on the optimum schedules for self-monitoring of blood pressure: a qualitative focus group and interview study. Br J Gen Pract. 2016;66:e819–30.
10. Little P, Barnett J, Barnsley L, Marjoram J, Fitzgerald-Barron A, Mant D. Comparison of acceptability of and preferences for different methods of measuring blood pressure in primary care. BMJ. 2002;325:258–9.
11. Logan AG, Dunai A, McIsaac WJ, Irvine MJ, Tisler A. Attitudes of primary care physicians and their patients about home blood pressure monitoring in Ontario. J Hypertens. 2008;26:446–52.
12. McGowan N, Padfield PL. Self blood pressure monitoring: a worthy substitute for ambulatory blood pressure? J Hum Hypertens. 2010;24:801–6.
13. Nasothimiou EG, Karpettas N, Dafni MG, Stergiou GS. Patients' preference for ambulatory versus home blood pressure monitoring. J Hum Hypertens. 2014;28:224–9.
14. Kronish IM, Kent S, Moise N, Shimbo D, Safford MM, Kynerd RE, et al. Barriers to conducting ambulatory and home blood pressure monitoring during hypertension screening in the United States. J Am Soc Hypertens. 2017;11:573–80.
15. Steinmann WC, Chitima-Matsiga R, Bagree S. What are specialist and primary care Clinicians' attitudes and practices regarding home blood pressure monitoring for hypertensive patients? Mo Med. 2011;108:433–47.

16. Tisler A, Dunai A, Keszei A, Fekete B, Othmane Tel H, Torzsa P, et al. Primary-care physicians' views about the use of home/self blood pressure monitoring: nationwide survey in Hungary. J Hypertens. 2006;24:1729–35.
17. Tsakiri C, Stergiou GS, Boivin JM. Implementation of home blood pressure monitoring in clinical practice. Clin Exp Hypertens. 2013;35:558–62.
18. Myers MG, Stergiou GS. Reporting bias: Achilles' heel of home blood pressure monitoring. J Am Soc Hypertens. 2014;8:350–7.
19. Parati G, Dolan E, McManus RJ, Omboni S. Home blood pressure telemonitoring in the 21st century. J Clin Hypertens (Greenwich). 2018;20:1128–32.
20. Uhlig K, Patel K, Ip S, Kitsios GD, Balk EM. Self-measured blood pressure monitoring in the management of hypertension: a systematic review and meta-analysis. Ann Intern Med. 2013;159:185–94.
21. Reboussin DM, Allen NB, Griswold ME, Guallar E, Hong Y, Lackland DT, et al. Systematic review for the 2017 ACC/AHA/AAPA/ABC/ACPM/AGS/APhA/ASH/ASPC/NMA/PCNA guideline for the prevention, detection, evaluation, and Management of High Blood Pressure in adults: a report of the American College of Cardiology/American Heart Association Task Force on Clinical Practice Guidelines. Circulation. 2018;138:e595–616.
22. Fletcher BR, Hinton L, Hartmann-Boyce J, Roberts NW, Bobrovitz N, McManus RJ. Self-monitoring blood pressure in hypertension, patient and provider perspectives: a systematic review and thematic synthesis. Patient Educ Couns. 2016;99:210–9.
23. Soghikian K, Casper SM, Fireman BH, Hunkeler EM, Hurley LB, Tekawa IS, et al. Home blood pressure monitoring. Effect on use of medical services and medical care costs. Med Care. 1992;30:855–65.
24. Billups SJ, Moore LR, Olson KL, Magid DJ. Cost-effectiveness evaluation of a home blood pressure monitoring program. Am J Manag Care. 2014;20:e380–7.
25. Fukunaga H, Ohkubo T, Kobayashi M, Tamaki Y, Kikuya M, Obara T, et al. Cost-effectiveness of the introduction of home blood pressure measurement in patients with office hypertension. J Hypertens. 2008;26:685–90.
26. Arrieta A, Woods JR, Qiao N, Jay SJ. Cost-benefit analysis of home blood pressure monitoring in hypertension diagnosis and treatment: an insurer perspective. Hypertension. 2014;64:891–6.
27. Lovibond K, Jowett S, Barton P, Caulfield M, Heneghan C, Hobbs FD, et al. Cost-effectiveness of options for the diagnosis of high blood pressure in primary care: a modelling study. Lancet. 2011;378:1219–30.
28. Beyhaghi H, Viera AJ. Comparative cost-effectiveness of clinic, home, or ambulatory blood pressure measurement for hypertension diagnosis in US adults. Hypertension. 2019;73(1):121–31.
29. Hodgkinson J, Mant J, Martin U, Guo B, Hobbs FD, Deeks JJ, et al. Relative effectiveness of clinic and home blood pressure monitoring compared with ambulatory blood pressure monitoring in diagnosis of hypertension: systematic review. BMJ. 2011;342:d3621.

Home Blood Pressure Monitoring in Clinical Research

10

Angeliki Ntineri, Kazuomi Kario, Ji-Guang Wang, William White, and George S. Stergiou

10.1 Introduction

The important role of out-of-office blood pressure (BP) monitoring has made home (HBPM) and ambulatory monitoring (ABPM) useful in the optimal diagnosis and management of hypertension. In contrast, conventional office BP measurements have limitations that may affect the precision of BP findings in clinical trials. This chapter presents the characteristics of HBPM that render it a useful tool in the design and conduct of clinical trials and how they can be applied in hypertension research (Table 10.1) [1–8].

A. Ntineri · G. S. Stergiou (✉)
Hypertension Center STRIDE-7, National and Kapodistrian University of Athens, School of Medicine, Third Department of Medicine, Sotiria Hospital, Athens, Greece
e-mail: gstergi@med.uoa.gr

K. Kario
Division of Cardiovascular Medicine, Department of Medicine, Jichi Medical University School of Medicine (JMU), Tochigi, Japan
e-mail: kkario@jichi.ac.jp

J.-G. Wang
The Shanghai Institute of Hypertension, Ruijin Hospital, Shanghai Jiaotong University School of Medicine, Shanghai, China

W. White
Calhoun Cardiology Center, University of Connecticut School of Medicine, Farmington, CT, USA
e-mail: wwhite@uchc.edu

Table 10.1 Characteristics of home compared to office and ambulatory blood pressure for clinical research (modified with permission from [1])

	Home BP	Office BP	Ambulatory BP
Number of BP measurements	++	+	+++
Misleading phenomena (white-coat effect, masked hypertension effect, placebo effect)	−	+	−
Observer bias elimination	+++ (automated devices or telemonitoring)	+	+++
Reproducibility	+++	+	+++
Study power and sample size	+++	+	+++
Subjects selection	+++	+	+++
Diagnosis of true resistant hypertension	++	+	+++
Assessment of treatment-induced BP changes	++	+	+++
Assessment of treatment-induced changes in organ damage	++	+	+++
Assessment of morning hypertension	+++	+	+++
Assessment of nocturnal hypertension	++ (specific devices)	−	+++
Assessment of variability			
– Short-term	−	−	++
– Mid-term	++	−	−
– Long-term	++	++	−
Association with preclinical organ damage	+++	+	+++
Association with cardiovascular events risk	+++	+	+++
Compliance with drug treatment	+++	+	+
Patients' preference	+++	+	+
Guidance in hypertension management	++	+	++
Repeated monitoring in longitudinal trials	+++	++	+
Cost-effectiveness	+++	++	+

BP blood pressure, + Superior, − Inferior

10.2 Advantages of HBPM for Clinical Research

HBPM has major advantages in clinical research. As with ABPM, HBPM provides multiple readings in the individual's usual environment. However, home measurements may be obtained over several days, weeks, or even months, whereas ABPM is typically conducted during a 24-h period and cannot be repeated more frequently than 2 or 3 times in a trial. On the contrary, office BP monitoring (OBPM) obtains a few readings, typically taken in the clinical environment which is a potentially stressful setting that promotes the emergence of the white-coat effect, masked hypertension, placebo effect, and observer bias [2]. Hence, HBPM and ABPM have advantages that result in superior reproducibility and diagnostic accuracy compared to conventional office BP measurements [3]. Regarding prognostic significance, HBPM has demonstrated close associations with several manifestations of early target organ damage and cardiovascular events risk, which are superior to those obtained by OBPM and similar to those by ABPM [4, 5]. In addition, HBPM is more acceptable to patients than ABPM, since it causes only minimal restriction of daily activities and no interruptions during sleep [6]. HBPM has been also shown to improve patients' compliance with drug treatment and hypertension control rates [2].

10.3   Implications of HBPM in Clinical Research

10.3.1 Selection of Study Participants

The selection of appropriate study participants is one of the most important methodological issues in clinical hypertension research. HBPM is a valuable diagnostic tool that accurately defines hypertension phenotypes in studies aiming to investigate the prevalence, characteristics, determinants, and prognostic significance of a specific BP pattern. In addition, isolation of BP patterns such as white-coat and masked hypertension that may exhibit heterogenous behavior and distort findings of a study is needed by out-of-office monitoring. For example, in study participants with white-coat hypertension, there is often minimal ambulatory BP response to antihypertensive drug therapy compared to those subjects with sustained hypertension [9]. Studies in patients with resistant hypertension also have demonstrated the importance of using HBPM for the reliable diagnosis and the exclusion of the white-coat hypertension phenomenon, which is common even among treated and moderately to severely hypertensive subjects [10, 11].

10.3.2 Improvement of Study Power and Reduction of Sample Size

The reproducibility of a BP measurement method, expressed as the standard deviation of differences between repeated measurements, plays a major role in the calculation of the sample size required for a clinical trial. As has been observed with ABPM, HBPM also has superior reproducibility to OBPM which makes it useful for clinical trials that compare the efficacy of antihypertensive drugs since it allows the same antihypertensive effect size to be identified with higher precision [3]. In other words, HBPM allows a smaller sample size to be recruited in order to identify a difference in the BP lowering effect of two drugs with the same study power [3, 12].

Based on power curves of a randomized crossover clinical trial comparing the antihypertensive efficacy of two drugs using clinic, ambulatory, or home BP measurements, for a trial aiming to detect a difference in the hypotensive effect of 10 mmHg for systolic BP, 5 mmHg for diastolic BP, or 3 mmHg for pulse pressure, the statistical power is much higher with HBPM and ABPM than with OBPM (Fig. 10.1) [13].

10.3.3 Evaluation of the Effects of Antihypertensive Drugs

10.3.3.1   Evaluation of the Magnitude of BP Lowering Effect

Because of its superior reproducibility to OBPM, HBPM provides a more accurate classification of the true baseline BP and improves the precision for the

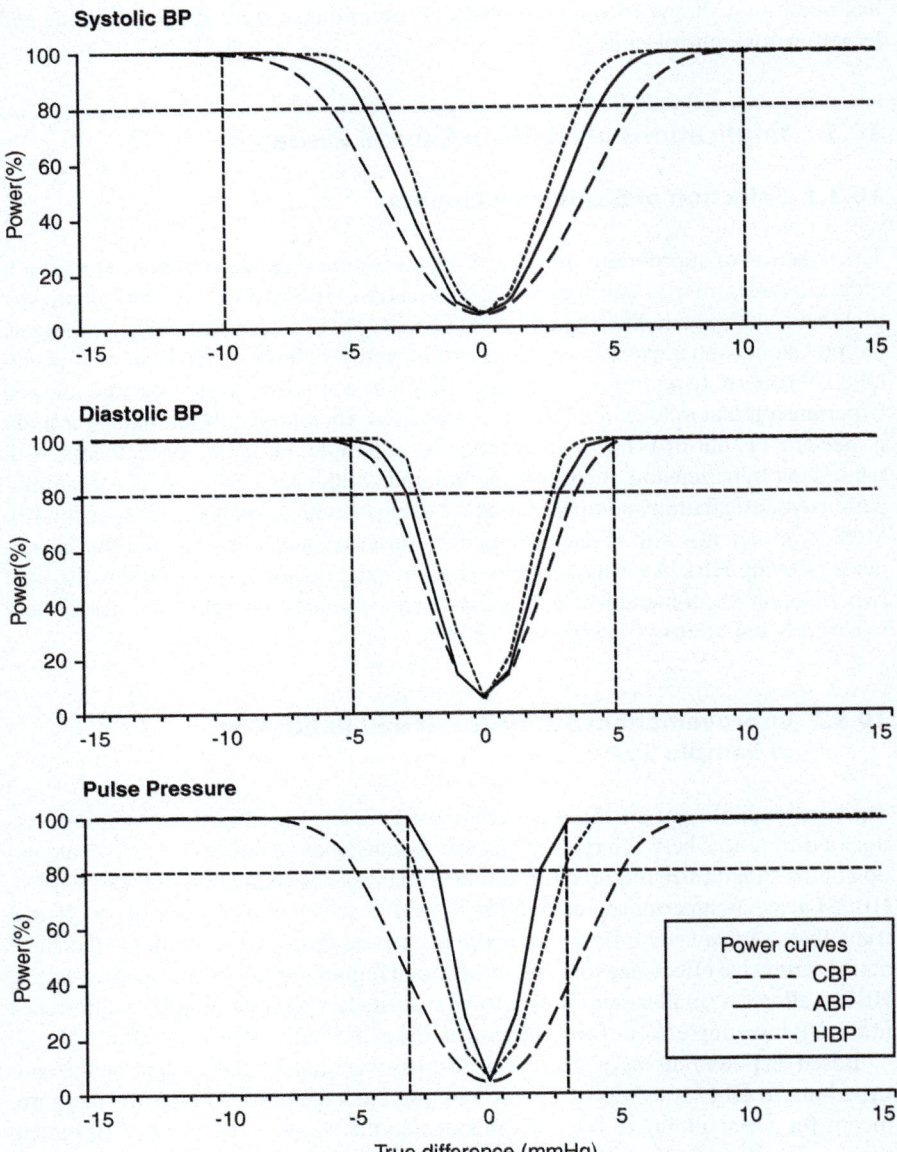

Fig. 10.1 Study power curves of a randomized crossover clinical trial comparing the efficacy of two antihypertensive drugs using blood pressure measurements in the clinic, at home and with ambulatory monitoring (from [13]). *BP* blood pressure, *CBP* clinic BP, *ABP* 24-h ambulatory BP, *HBP* home BP. Horizontal dotted lines indicate 80% power to detect a difference in the hypotensive effect of the drugs of 10 mmHg for systolic, 5 mmHg for diastolic BP, or 3 mmHg for pulse pressure (vertical dotted lines)

determination of antihypertensive drug treatment-induced BP changes. These benefits are also related to the absence of the placebo effect, regression dilution bias (regression to the mean), and observer bias (when electronic devices with automated memory are used), which typically affect clinical trials when OBPM is employed.

In a randomized controlled parallel-group design study which evaluated the antihypertensive efficacy of the angiotensin-converting enzyme inhibitor trandolapril versus placebo, HBPM, but not OBPM, determined the expected antihypertensive effect of trandolapril versus placebo [14]. Another clinical trial comparing the 24-h efficacy of beta-blocker bisoprolol with the calcium channel blocker nitrendipine found no difference in the antihypertensive effect of the two drugs when clinic or daytime ABP were used, whereas home and nighttime ambulatory BP measurements detected a greater systolic BP fall with bisoprolol [12]. Furthermore, a randomized crossover clinical trial comparing the BP lowering effect of the angiotensin-converting enzyme inhibitor lisinopril with the angiotensin receptor blocker losartan reported that all the BP measurement methods (clinic, ambulatory, and home) demonstrated greater efficacy with lisinopril (Fig. 10.2) with HBPM providing the greatest precision ($p < 0.001$ versus $p < 0.01$ for 24-hour ABPM and $p < 0.05$ for OBPM) [13]. Home and ambulatory BP, but not office BP, detected the antihypertensive effect of lisinopril on pulse pressure (Fig. 10.2) [13]. Regarding comparative assessment of the antihypertensive effect of drug combinations versus monotherapy, a study by Mancia et al. showed that a calcium channel blocker/angiotensin-converting enzyme inhibitor combination was more effective in lowering home BP vs. monotherapy with these drugs or placebo [15].

HBPM has also been used to investigate the BP lowering effects of non-antihypertensive drugs such as the sodium-glucose co-transporter 2 (SGLT-2) inhibitor canagliflozin in order to explain the beneficial role in cardiovascular risk via potential pleiotropic actions in patients with poorly controlled diabetes and nocturnal BP [16].

10.3.3.2 Evaluation of the Duration of Action of Antihypertensive Drugs

The smoothness and consistency of 24-h efficacy by an antihypertensive drug are usually assessed by the trough-to-peak ratio (T/P), which is an index produced from 24-h ambulatory or with repeated clinic BP measurements. Alternatively, HBPM that obtains measurements before drug intake and post-dose can provide information on the "trough" and "plateau" (not peak) effect calculating the morning-to-evening (M/E) home BP ratio [17, 18]. A randomized controlled trial showed both T/P and M/E BP ratios to be higher with lisinopril compared to losartan, which was consistent in a sensitivity analysis conducted only in drug responders (Fig. 10.3) [17]. The difference between morning and evening home BP values (morning-evening difference) was shown to be associated with cardiac damage in a study of untreated hypertensive patients by Matsui et al. [19].

While the M/E home BP ratio may fail to identify an excessive hypotensive effect at peak, the velocity of the antihypertensive effect and time of maximum efficacy (stabilization time) can be evaluated by HBPM using an exponential decay function analysis based on serial home BP measurements [20, 21].

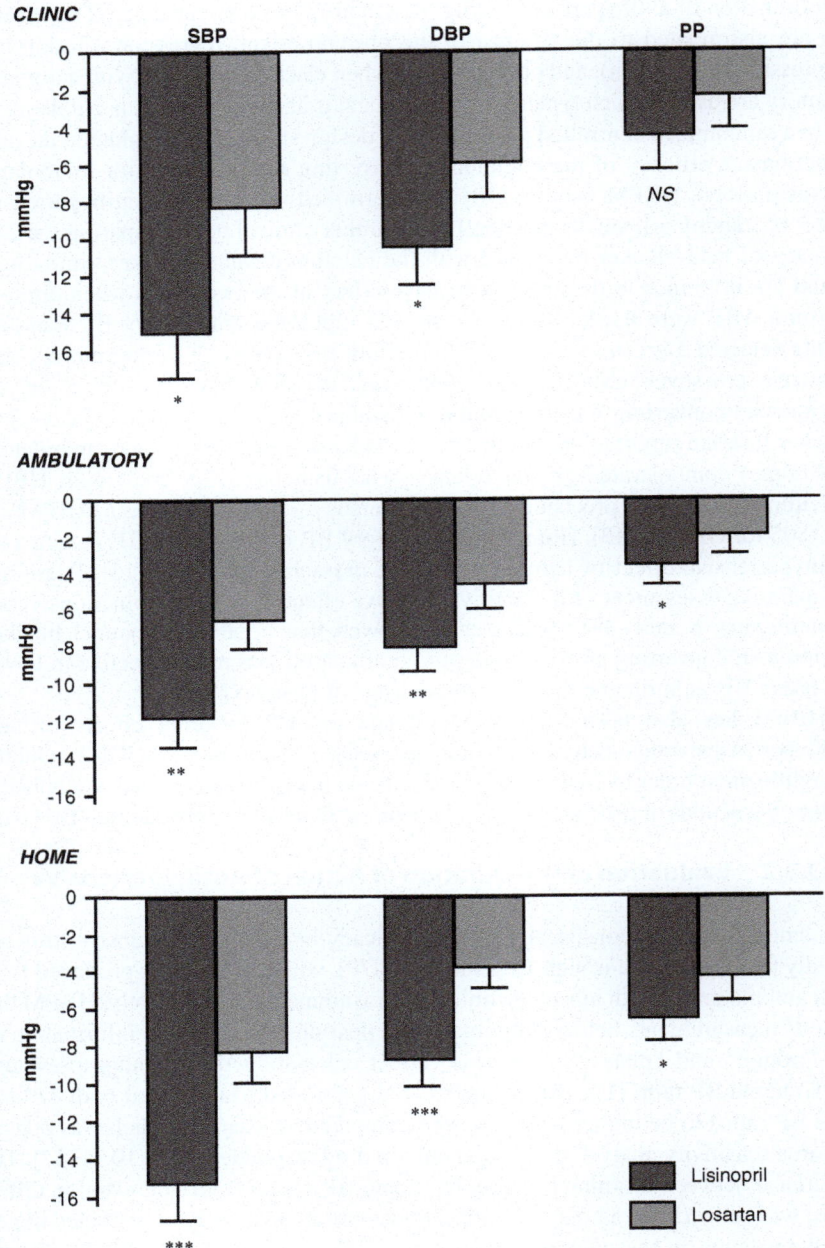

Fig. 10.2 Randomized crossover comparative clinical trial of the effects of two antihypertensive drugs on clinic, 24-h ambulatory and home blood pressure (from [13]). *SBP* systolic blood pressure, *DBP* diastolic blood pressure, *PP* pulse pressure, ∗, P < 0.05; ∗∗, P < 0.01; ∗∗∗, P < 0.001 for differences between the two drugs)

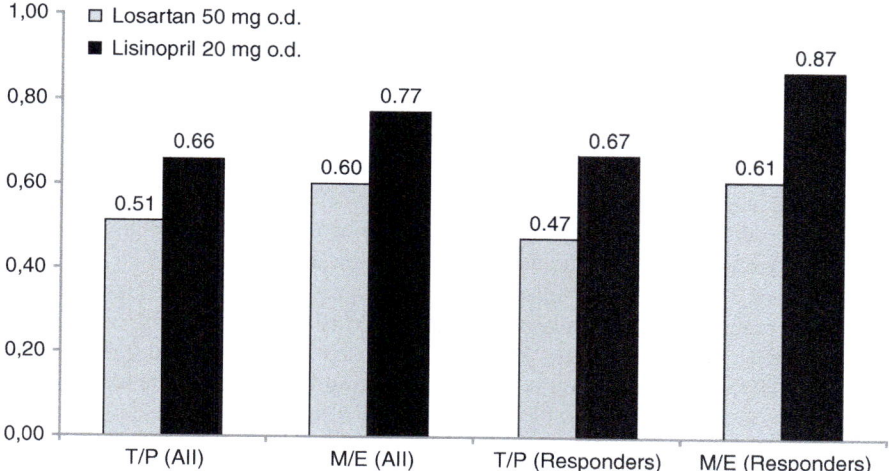

Fig. 10.3 Morning-to-evening (M/E) home blood pressure ratio versus trough-to-peak (T/P) ambulatory blood pressure ratio for assessing the duration of antihypertensive effect of two drugs in all study subjects and in those who responded to treatment (modified with permission from [17])

10.3.3.3   Chronotherapy in Hypertension

Chronotherapy studies have utilized HBPM to explore the optimal time of drug administration in relation to BP levels, organ damage and adverse effects. Using HBPM, Mori et al. showed that olmesartan effectively decreased morning home BP, regardless of the time of drug administration [22]. Moreover, Mengden et al. found that HBPM, but not OBPM or ABPM, determined the pharmacodynamic effects of the timing of dosing of once daily amlodipine on 24-h BP control (greater BP reductions for morning than for evening administration) [23]. However, when the analysis accounted for the poorer drug compliance of evening versus morning administration, HBPM also did not detect a BP difference. Hashimoto et al. reported that bedtime administration of the centrally acting alpha$_2$-agonists guanabenz and clonidine effectively suppressed morning hypertension as assessed with home BP measurements [24]. Finally, a study exploring the dosing time of the angiotensin II receptor blocker candesartan titrated by self-measured HBPM on cardiorenal damage in patients with hypertension showed that bedtime was superior to morning dosing for reducing microalbuminuria, whereas there were no differences in the reduction of BP levels [25].

10.3.4   Assessment of Drug-Induced Effects on Organ Damage and Cardiovascular Events

Clinical trials designed to associate regression of target organ damage and BP changes induced by antihypertensive treatment initiation or modification require long-term follow-up for the beneficial effects on the heart, the arteries, and the kidneys to be apparent. HBPM seems the most convenient tool for both researchers and participants to reliably track BP changes during longer time periods and show their clinical relevance with lower monitoring costs. A study with 13.4 months follow-up demonstrated that treatment-induced changes in home or ambulatory BP were more closely related than office BP with changes in indices of heart, vascular, and renal organ damage [26]. However, another study with 1-year follow-up reported that treatment-induced regression in left ventricular hypertrophy was more closely associated with ambulatory BP effects and far less with home BP, and unrelated to office BP changes [27]. A limitation of this study was that only two home readings were obtained, which could have had a substantial impact on the reliability of the home BP data.

In the last 20 years, hypertension outcome trials starting from the Hypertension Optimal Treatment (HOT) study have used HBPM [28]. The Home blood pressure measurement with Olmesartan Naive patients to Establish Standard Target blood pressure (HONEST) study investigated the morning home BP threshold related to increased risk of major cardiovascular events over a 2-year follow-up in participants treated with an angiotensin receptor blocker based regimen, even if they had controlled office BP [29].

10.3.5 Evaluation of Drug-Induced Effects on Blood Pressure Variability

Home BP measurements allow for the investigation of differential effects of antihypertensive drugs on intermediate-term and day-by-day BP variability. Studies have shown that treatment with beta-blockers exacerbates, whereas alpha-blockers lower home BP variability [30]. Another study showed that participants treated with an angiotensin receptor blocker had higher systolic home BP variability compared to those on a calcium channel blocker [31]. Moreover, the addition of a calcium channel blocker on an angiotensin receptor blocker was shown to decrease home BP variability more than the addition of a thiazide [32]. In contrast, recent findings from the HOMED-BP study comparing monotherapy with calcium channel blockers, angiotensin-converting enzyme inhibitors, or angiotensin receptor blockers for effects on changes in home BP variability in newly treated hypertensive patients suggested that the magnitude of BP variability reduction did not differ by antihypertensive drug classes [33].

HBPM can explore the prognostic significance of the intermediate- and long-term BP variability, a parameter which is currently felt to be independently associated with common study endpoints including subclinical target organ damage or cardiovascular events and mortality [30]. Hence, it has been hypothesized that treatment-induced changes in home BP variability could also be associated with cardiovascular endpoints. Matsui et al. reported an independent association between a change in pulse wave velocity with corresponding change in systolic home BP variability achieved using an angiotensin receptor blocker/calcium channel blocker combination, whereas another study showed that the decrease in albuminuria was not associated with that of home BP variability after treatment with an angiotensin receptor blocker/thiazide combination [32, 34]. In contrast, in the HOMED-BP study, although baseline evening (but not morning) home BP variability predicted major cardiovascular endpoints independently of BP level, home BP variability after monotherapy had no predictive power for cardiovascular outcome [33].

10.3.6 Assessment of Other Aspects of Home Blood Pressure Profile and Behavior

10.3.6.1 Morning Blood Pressure
Studies have shown that morning hypertension has independent prognostic significance for target organ damage and stroke [35]. HBMP and ABPM appear to be interchangeable methods for the assessment of morning hypertension with close diagnostic agreement [36]. HBPM could be regarded more attractive for this assessment, since morning readings at home are taken under more standardized conditions in terms of environment, physical activity and body posture and at trough level of drug action, and could be assessed over several days or weeks. In treated patients, the home BP measurements are taken before drug intake, and hence are trough measurements [37]. Two important studies used HBPM to explore the effect of angiotensin II receptor antagonists on morning BP and reported beneficial results [38, 39].

10.3.6.2 Nocturnal Blood Pressure
Evidence suggests that, compared to other aspects of the BP profile, nocturnal BP is an independent and strong predictor of cardiovascular risk. Novel low-cost home monitors allow automated nighttime BP monitoring on different days. There is evidence that nocturnal HBPM yields reproducible BP values [40]. A recent review and meta-analysis concluded that nocturnal home BP had similar values and close correlation with nighttime ambulatory BP with close agreement in detecting non-dippers and comparable associations with indices of preclinical target-organ damage [41]. The above features suggest that nocturnal HBPM may become an attractive low-cost alternative to ambulatory monitoring for the evaluation of nocturnal hypertension, detection of non-dippers, and the assessment of treatment-induced changes in nocturnal BP in clinical trials.

10.3.6.3 Blood Pressure Dynamics
HBPM has been successfully applied for tracking specific BP changes during usual activities or interventions. Postprandial hypotension, a risk factor for cardiovascular disease, can be detected through home BP measurements before and after meals, a characteristic that may make ABPM redundant especially if the test is being used for screening for asymptomatic conditions [42]. HBPM was recently reported to be a suitable alternative for ABPM for monitoring BP reduction after renal denervation. The fact that BP changes were gradual and lasted at least one year after the intervention highlights the usefulness of HBPM in such projects because of its greater availability, low cost, and patients' acceptance for frequent use [43].

10.4   How to Use HBPM in Clinical Research

Optimal application of HBPM in clinical trials is of paramount importance for gathering reliable results. The necessary equipment includes electronic (oscillometric) upper-arm cuff devices that have been successfully validated using an established protocol with cuffs of appropriate size for study participants' arm circumference (www.stridebp.org) [2]. The BP monitors should also be equipped with automated memory or PC link capacity or telemonitoring systems to prevent "reporting bias" (over- or under-reporting of self-measurements by patients) and secure a reliable evaluation of BP [2]. Participants should be trained in the measurement of home BP and the proper use of the devices. Measurements should take place in a quiet room after 5-min of rest in the seated position with back supported and arm resting at heart level [2]. The monitoring schedule as recommended by current guidelines require duplicate (with a 1 min interval) morning (before drug intake if treated) and evening measurements for 7 days (but no less than 3 days). The average of all readings should be evaluated after excluding those of the first day [2].

10.5   Conclusions

During the last two decades HBPM has been used increasingly in clinical hypertension research. Its multiple advantages lead to superior diagnostic reliability and measurement reproducibility, ensuring improved accuracy of clinical trials than when using office BP measurements and thereby leading to smaller sample size and lower research costs, together with better patients' acceptance, particularly for longer-term trials.

References

1. Stergiou GS, Ntineri A. Home (self) monitoring of blood pressure in clinical trials. In: White WB, editor. Blood pressure monitoring in cardiovascular medicine and therapeutics. Third edition. New York: Springer; 2016. https://doi.org/10.1007/978-3-319-22771-9.
2. Parati G, Stergiou GS, Asmar R, Bilo G, de Leeuw P, Imai Y, et al. European Society of Hypertension guidelines for blood pressure monitoring at home: a summary report of the second international consensus conference on home blood pressure monitoring. J Hypertens. 2008;26(8):1505–26.
3. Stergiou GS, Baibas NM, Gantzarou AP, Skeva II, Kalkana CB, Roussias LG, et al. Reproducibility of home, ambulatory, and clinic blood pressure: implications for the design of trials for the assessment of antihypertensive drug efficacy. Am J Hypertens. 2002;15(2 Pt 1):101–4.
4. Ward AM, Takahashi O, Stevens R, Heneghan C. Home measurement of blood pressure and cardiovascular disease: systematic review and meta-analysis of prospective studies. J Hypertens. 2012;30(3):449–56.
5. Bliziotis IA, Destounis A, Stergiou GS. Home versus ambulatory and office blood pressure in predicting target organ damage in hypertension: a systematic review and meta-analysis. J Hypertens. 2012;30(7):1289–99.

6. Nasothimiou EG, Karpettas N, Dafni MG, Stergiou GS. Patients' preference for ambulatory versus home blood pressure monitoring. J Hum Hypertens. 2014;28(4):224–9.

7. Asayama K, Ohkubo T, Metoki H, Obara T, Inoue R, Kikuya M, et al. Cardiovascular outcomes in the first trial of antihypertensive therapy guided by self-measured home blood pressure. Hypertens Res. 2012;35(11):1102–10.

8. Boubouchairopoulou N, Karpettas N, Athanasakis K, Kollias A, Protogerou AD, Achimastos A, et al. Cost estimation of hypertension management based on home blood pressure monitoring alone or combined office and ambulatory blood pressure measurements. J Am Soc Hypertens. 2014;8(10):732–8.

9. Mancia G, Facchetti R, Parati G, Zanchetti A. Effect of long-term antihypertensive treatment on white-coat hypertension. Hypertension. 2014;64(6):1388–98.

10. Nasothimiou EG, Tzamouranis D, Roussias LG, Stergiou GS. Home versus ambulatory blood pressure monitoring in the diagnosis of clinic resistant and true resistant hypertension. J Hum Hypertens. 2012;26(12):696–700.

11. Bhatt DL, Kandzari DE, O'Neill WW, D'Agostino R, Flack JM, Katzen BT, et al. A controlled trial of renal denervation for resistant hypertension. N Engl J Med. 2014;370(15):1393–401.

12. Mengden T, Binswanger B, Weisser B, Vetter W. An evaluation of self-measured blood pressure in a study with a calcium-channel antagonist versus a beta-blocker. Am J Hypertens. 1992;5(3):154–60.

13. Stergiou GS, Efstathiou SP, Skeva II, Baibas NM, Kalkana CB, Mountokalakis TD. Assessment of drug effects on blood pressure and pulse pressure using clinic, home and ambulatory measurements. J Hum Hypertens. 2002;16(10):729–35.

14. Vaur L, Dubroca II, Dutrey-Dupagne C, Genès N, Chatellier G, Bouvier-d'Yvoire M, et al. Superiority of home blood pressure measurements over office measurements for testing antihypertensive drugs. Blood Press Monit. 1998;3(2):107–14.

15. Mancia G, Omboni S, Chazova I, Coca A, Girerd X, Haller H, et al. Effects of the lercanidipine-enalapril combination vs. the corresponding monotherapies on home blood pressure in hypertension: evidence from a large database. J Hypertens. 2016;34(1):139–48.

16. Kario K, Hoshide S, Okawara Y, Tomitani N, Yamauchi K, Ohbayashi H, et al. Effect of canagliflozin on nocturnal home blood pressure in Japanese patients with type 2 diabetes mellitus: the SHIFT-J study. J Clin Hypertens (Greenwich). 2018;20(10):1527–35.

17. Stergiou GS, Efstathiou SP, Skeva II, Baibas NM, Roussias LG, Mountokalakis TD. Comparison of the smoothness index, the trough: peak ratio and the morning: evening ratio in assessing the features of the antihypertensive drug effect. J Hypertens. 2003;21(5):913–20.

18. Nishimura T, Hashimoto J, Ohkubo T, Kikuya M, Metoki H, Asayama K, et al. Efficacy and duration of action of the four selective angiotensin II subtype 1 receptor blockers, losartan, candesartan, valsartan and telmisartan, in patients with essential hypertension determined by home blood pressure measurements. Clin Exp Hypertens. 2005;27(6):477–89.

19. Matsui Y, Eguchi K, Shibasaki S, Shimizu M, Ishikawa J, Shimada K, et al. Association between the morning-evening difference in home blood pressure and cardiac damage in untreated hypertensive patients. J Hypertens. 2009;27(4):712–20.

20. Metoki H, Ohkubo T, Kikuya M, Asayama K, Inoue R, Obara T, et al. The velocity of antihypertensive effect of losartan/hydrochlorothiazide and angiotensin II receptor blocker. J Hypertens. 2012;30(7):1478–86.

21. Satoh M, Haga T, Hosaka M, Metoki H, Murakami T, et al. The velocity of antihypertensive effects of seven angiotensin II receptor blockers determined by home blood pressure measurements. J Hypertens. 2016;34(6):1218–23.

22. Mori H, Yamamoto H, Ukai H, Yuasa S, Nakajima K, Mikawa T, et al. Comparison of effects of angiotensin II receptor blocker on morning home blood pressure and cardiorenal protection between morning administration and evening administration in hypertensive patients: the COMPATIBLE study. Hypertens Res. 2013;36(3):202–7.

23. Mengden T, Binswanger B, Spühler T, Weisser B, Vetter W. The use of self-measured blood pressure determinations in assessing dynamics of drug compliance in a study with amlodipine once a day, morning versus evening. J Hypertens. 1993;11(12):1403–11.

24. Hashimoto J, Chonan K, Aoki Y, Ugajin T, Yamaguchi J, Nishimura T, et al. Therapeutic effects of evening administration of guanabenz and clonidine on morning hypertension: evaluation using home-based blood pressure measurements. J Hypertens. 2003;21(4):805–11.
25. Kario K, Hoshide S, Shimizu M, Yano Y, Eguchi K, Ishikawa J, et al. Effect of dosing time of angiotensin II receptor blockade titrated by self-measured blood pressure recordings on cardiorenal protection in hypertensives: the Japan morning surge-target organ protection (J-TOP) study. J Hypertens. 2010;28(7):1574–83.
26. Karpettas N, Destounis A, Kollias A, Nasothimiou E, Moyssakis I, Stergiou GS. Prediction of treatment-induced changes in target-organ damage using changes in clinic, home and ambulatory blood pressure. Hypertens Res. 2014;37(6):543–7.
27. Mancia G, Zanchetti A, Agabiti-Rosei E, Benemio G, De Cesaris R, Fogari R, et al. Ambulatory blood pressure is superior to clinic blood pressure in predicting treatment-induced regression of left ventricular hypertrophy. SAMPLE study group. Study on ambulatory monitoring of blood pressure and Lisinopril evaluation. Circulation. 1997;95(6):1464–70.
28. Kjeldsen SE, Hedner T, Jamerson K, Julius S, Haley WE, Zabalgoitia M, et al. Hypertension optimal treatment (HOT) study: home blood pressure in treated hypertensive subjects. Hypertension. 1998;31(4):1014–20.
29. Kario K, Saito I, Kushiro T, Teramukai S, Ishikawa Y, Mori Y, et al. Home blood pressure and cardiovascular outcomes in patients during antihypertensive therapy: primary results of HONEST, a large-scale prospective, real-world observational study. Hypertension. 2014;64(5):989–96.
30. Stergiou GS, Ntineri A, Kollias A, Ohkubo T, Imai Y, Parati G. Blood pressure variability assessed by home measurements: a systematic review. Hypertens Res. 2014;37(6):565–72.
31. Ishikura K, Obara T, Kato T, Kikuya M, Shibamiya T, Shinki T, et al. Associations between day-by-day variability in blood pressure measured at home and antihypertensive drugs: the J-HOME-morning study. Clin Exp Hypertens. 2012;34(4):297–304.
32. Matsui Y, O'Rourke MF, Hoshide S, Ishikawa J, Shimada K, Kario K. Combined effect of angiotensin II receptor blocker and either a calcium channel blocker or diuretic on day-by-day variability of home blood pressure: the Japan combined treatment with olmesartan and a calcium-channel blocker versus olmesartan and diuretics randomized efficacy study. Hypertension. 2012;59(6):1132–8.
33. Asayama K, Ohkubo T, Hanazawa T, Watabe D, Hosaka M, Satoh M, et al. Does antihypertensive drug class affect day-to-day variability of self-measured home blood pressure? The HOMED-BP study. J Am Heart Assoc. 2016;5(3):e002995.
34. Hoshide S, Yano Y, Shimizu M, Eguchi K, Ishikawa J, Kario K. Is home blood pressure variability itself an interventional target beyond lowering mean home blood pressure during antihypertensive treatment? Hypertens Res. 2012;35(8):862–6.
35. Asayama K, Ohkubo T, Kikuya M, Obara T, Metoki H, Inoue R, et al. Prediction of stroke by home "morning" versus "evening" blood pressure values: the Ohasama study. Hypertension. 2006;48(4):737–43.
36. Stergiou GS, Nasothimiou EG, Roussias LG. Morning hypertension assessed by home or ambulatory monitoring: different aspects of the same phenomenon? J Hypertens. 2010;28(9):1846–53.
37. Stergiou G, Parati G. Further insights into the 24-h blood pressure profile by home blood pressure monitoring: the issue of morning hypertension. J Hypertens. 2009;27(4):696–9.
38. Redon J, Bilo G, Parati G, Surge Steering Committee. The effects of telmisartan alone or in combination with hydrochlorothiazide on morning home blood pressure control: the SURGE 2 practice-based study. Blood Press. 2013;22(6):377–85.
39. Kario K, Saito I, Kushiro T, Teramukai S, Ishikawa Y, Hiramatsu K, et al. Effect of the angiotensin II receptor antagonist olmesartan on morning home blood pressure in hypertension: HONEST study at 16 weeks. J Hum Hypertens. 2013;27(12):721–8.
40. Asayama K, Fujiwara T, Hoshide S, Ohkubo T, Kario K, Stergiou GS, et al. Nocturnal blood pressure measured by home devices: evidence and perspective for clinical application. J Hypertens. 2019;37(5):905–16.

41. Kollias A, Ntineri A, Stergiou GS. Association of night-time home blood pressure with night-time ambulatory blood pressure and target-organ damage: a systematic review and meta-analysis. J Hypertens. 2017;35(3):442–52.

42. Alfie J. Utility of home blood pressure monitoring to evaluate postprandial blood pressure in treated hypertensive patients. Ther Adv Cardiovasc Dis. 2015;9(4):133–9.

43. Beeftink MM, Spiering W, Bots ML, Verloop WL, De Jager RL, Sanders MF, et al. Renal denervation in a real life setting: a gradual decrease in home blood pressure. PLoS One. 2016;11(9):e0162251.

Home Blood Pressure Telemonitoring: Conventional Approach and Perspectives from Mobile Health Technology

11

Gianfranco Parati, Juan Eugenio Ochoa, Nicolas Postel-Vinay, Dario Pellegrini, Camilla Torlasco, Stefano Omboni, and Richard J. McManus

11.1 Introduction

Home blood pressure monitoring (HBPM) represents a cost-effective and well-validated strategy for out-of-office BP monitoring [1]. In consideration of its well-known advantages (i.e., superior prognostic value against conventional clinic BP

G. Parati (✉)
Department of Medicine and Surgery, University of Milano-Bicocca, Milan, Italy

Istituto Auxologico Italiano, IRCCS, Department of Cardiovascular, Neural and Metabolic Sciences, Milan, Italy
e-mail: gianfranco.parati@unimib.it

J. E. Ochoa · D. Pellegrini · C. Torlasco
Department of Cardiovascular Neural and Metabolic Sciences, Istituto Auxologico Italiano, IRCCS, Milan, Italy
e-mail: c.torlasco@auxologico.it

N. Postel-Vinay
Hypertension Unit ESH Excellence Center, Hôpital Européen Georges-Pompidou, Paris, France
e-mail: nicolas.postel-vinay@aphp.fr

S. Omboni
Clinical Research Unit, Italian Institute of Telemedicine, Solbiate Arno, Varese, Italy

Scientifc Research Department of Cardiology, Sechenov First Moscow State Medical University, Moscow, Russian Federation
e-mail: stefano.omboni@iitelemed.org

R. J. McManus
Nuffield Department of Primary Care Health Sciences, University of Oxford, Oxford, UK
e-mail: richard.mcmanus@phc.ox.ac.uk

levels, easy availability, and good acceptance by patients) most hypertension guidelines have recommend the use of HBPM as a useful method for the evaluation of patients with suspected or diagnosed and treated hypertension [2, 3]. Despite its demonstrated benefits, a critical aspect for a proper application of HBPM in clinical practice is data reporting by patients and their interpretation by practicing physicians. In general, BP values obtained by patients at home are reported in handwritten logbooks which sometimes are inaccurate and/or illegible making interpretation of HBPM values difficult. This may discourage physicians from using HBPM data for clinical decision making. A possible solution to this problem was the introduction of HBP measuring devices equipped with memory. However, also in this case the problems of reporting may persist since data could be stored over different time periods in different devices. Alternatively, BP measurements taken from different family members could be stored in the same device memory log, with the risk of having average family BP levels rather than individual BP values. A potentially better solution has been provided more recently by progress in information and communication technologies, which in the last decades have made possible the remote transmission of BP values, measured at home or in a community setting, to the doctor's office or hospital, by means of telehealth strategies, an approach defined as home BP telemonitoring (HBPT). The conventional approach to HBPT has been based on the use of strategies based on computer-tailored interventions through the Internet (see Fig. 11.1) and a number of observational and randomized controlled studies have shown its efficacy in improving patients' compliance and adherence to antihypertensive treatment and in achieving more satisfactory hypertension control rates, thus improving cardiovascular protection by preventing the adverse consequences associated with elevated BP levels [4, 5]. In recent years, the widespread use of smartphone technologies, along with the development of applications for BP monitoring and remote transmission, has offered a new approach to HBPT (mHealth). Although, a number of issues, mainly related to the scientific validation of applications developed for mobile healthcare support, still need to be addressed, preliminary data from small studies have

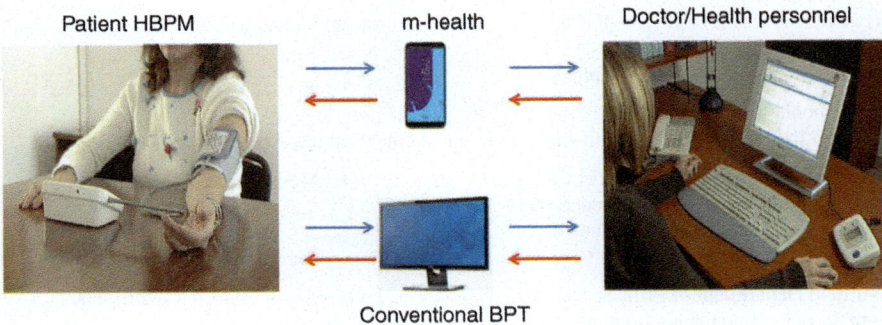

Fig. 11.1 Home Blood Pressure Telemonitoring: conventional and mobile health-based approaches

suggested the value of these technologies in improving patients' compliance and adherence to antihypertensive treatment, and in achieving higher BP control rates [6]. This chapter will review the role of BPT in hypertension management, focusing on the reasons for its development, the methodological aspects that should be considered for its clinical implementation as well as its role in improving hypertension control and cardiovascular risk reduction. Current evidence on the use of mobile applications for the management of hypertension will also be addressed by highlighting their potential for clinical use, the current limitations and the yet pending issues to be addressed in future studies.

11.2 Definitions

Telemedicine or telehealth consists in the exchange or delivery of medical information (e.g., health parameters, biological signals, diagnostic images) from one site to another via electronic communications in order to provide diagnosis and care at distance [7].

For many years, telemedicine systems were based mainly on strategies in which teletransmission was performed by means of personal computers equipped with internet connection [8]. However, the worldwide increase in the use of smartphones observed in recent years, along with the development of applications for patients' data monitoring, has offered new perspectives for telemedicine and the potential to improve interaction between doctors and patients, an approach defined as **"mobile health" or m-health** [9–11]. BPT represents a particular application of telemedicine using either computer-tailored or m-health strategies [12]. It consists of automatic data transmission of BP values and additional parameters, from the patient's living site (home or work place HBPT) or from a professional healthcare environment (e.g., primary care clinic or community pharmacy) to the doctor's office or to a hospital [12] (Box 11.1).

Box 11.1: Definitions
e-health of Digital health
The use of electronic processes and information and communication technologies to provide healthcare services
Telemedicine (also referred to as telehealth)
Teletransmission of health-related data from one site to another via electronic communications
M-health or "mobile health"
Teletransmission of health-related data by means of mobile communication devices (i.e., smartphones)
Blood Pressure Telemonitoring (BPT)
Teletransmission of BP values by means of traditional computer-based or m-health strategies

11.3 Methodological Aspects for Application of BPT

11.3.1 Conventional (eHealth Based) BPT Systems

The wide availability and low cost of automated BP measuring devices, the current advances in communication and information technologies, and the emphasis put by healthcare systems on delivering patient-centered care have stimulated development of home BPT, i.e., a particular application of telemedicine based on either personal computer or m-health strategies (see Fig. 11.1 and Box 11.1).

Devices for home BPT are usually based on automated upper-arm BP monitors which may collect multiple readings either over the 24-h, when applying 24 h ambulatory BP monitoring, or during several days, when repeated self BP measurements are performed by patients at home. Given the large number of monitors commercially available, significant differences among them may be observed in terms of data collection, transmission, reporting and reminders (for BP measurement to be performed and/or for medication intake). A list of available technologies for BP measurement, collection, and teletransmission is presented in Table 11.1.

Overall, home BPT systems require active involvement of patients who should self-monitor their BP levels and other related clinical variables and send these values to a healthcare provider. Current HBPT solutions allow self-BP measurements performed by patients at home to be in the device memory and the forwarded, immediately or periodically, to a remote computer host through a landline broadband or mobile network, and through the web by applying encryption transmission protocols which ensure data integrity and security [13]. Once data are received at the central telemedicine server they are stored and analyzed. Reports are automatically generated and then reviewed by a healthcare professional (usually a technician, a nurse, or a pharmacist), before they are submitted to the reporting physician, although in some instances reports are directly sent to the family doctor in charge. At the end of this process a medical report is forwarded to the patient and referring primary physician through a website, via e-mail or through dedicated smartphone apps (see Fig. 11.1). During all these processes the healthcare professional may also interact with the patient in order to obtain feedbacks on his/her health status and adjust treatment according to the indications of the managing physician (co-intervention or additional support) [14].

11.3.2 mHealth-Based BPT Strategies

As shown in Table 11.2, mHealth-based HBPT strategies can be implemented using different types of smartphone applications (Apps) currently available. **Apps that record and store BP values manually inserted by users** are the simplest ones, as they only require the user to manually enter the BP values he or she has detected with a measurement device. The main advantages of these apps are flexibility and

Table 11.1 Types of BP measuring devices and data collection and communication technologies used for blood pressure telemonitoring

BP measuring devices
- Automated devices (wired or wireless)
- Multiple parameters monitoring devices (e.g., single channel ECG, pulse oximetry, body temperature, blood glucose, medication intake) also known as "medical tricorders"
- Wireless smartphone applications (paired with an external wireless BP monitor or turning the smartphone into a cuffless BPM device)
- Wearable monitors for long-term surveillance (e.g., wrist tonometers or finger pletismographs)

Data communication technologies
Data transmission (download) from the device
- Dedicated wireless devices based on bluetooth, wi-fi, zigbee or NFC and with built-in mobile phone-based transmission systems (e.g., home hubs or smart boxes)
- Handheld devices (smartphones, tablets, PDAs, etc.) with wireless communication linked to private (home) or public (community) wi-fi access points or to the mobile public network
- Desktop or laptop computers linked to the BP measuring devices via wired (USB cable) or wireless connection

Data transmission (upload) to the telemedicine provider
- Landline broadband wired telephone lines (via a data modem or an acoustic coupling system)
- Broadband mobile network
- Peer-to-peer connection or the Internet
- Health exchange servers acting as single point forward hubs in the cloud (gateway)

Type of data transmitted
- Immediate or periodic automatic forward of encrypted data strings with proprietary or standard formats
- Manual data input by text messaging (SMS, social media applications such as whatsapp, facebook messenger, etc.)
- E-mail messaging (manual data input or list of readings sent as an attachment)
- Website with dedicated forms allowing manual data input or manual upload of files

Adapted by permission from Parati et al. [14]. *BP* blood pressure, *ECG* electrocardiogram, *NFC* near field communication, *PDA* personal digital assistant, *USB* universal serial bus, *SMS* short text messaging

availability, as they do not require the measurements to be performed at the same time of data entry, and they are not tied to a single device type. Thus, measurements can be performed at any time and with any device of choice. The consequent critical (and obvious) drawback is the consistent risk of errors during transcription of measured BP values into the app.

Apps associated to automated transmission of BP values from the BP measurement devices to the phone have the advantage to be associated to either conventional or automated oscillometric BP measurement devices able to send data to smartphones, or equipped with specifically designed cuffs with an inflating system that works only when paired to a phone. Although wireless cuffs that work with a paired phone have been developed and seem appealing for the user due to their extreme portability, their accuracy has been questioned due to the high variability of BP measures compared to standard BP measurement techniques [15].

Table 11.2 Main mobile phone applications for mHealth-based BPT strategies

Type of App	Advantages	Disadvantages
Manual insertion of BP values by user	– Flexibility – Widely available in digital stores – Not tied to specific devices – Measurement and recording of BP values can be performed at different times – May provide adaptative self-care practices via text messaging	– High risk of errors in transcription of BP values from the device to the phone
Automated transmission from an oscillometric device to the phone	– Widely available – High accuracy of validated devices – Automated transmission of data: easy to obtain and low risk of errors	– Tied to a specific device brand or model – Cost
Wireless cuff paired to the phone	– High portability – Automated transmission of data: easy to obtain and low risk of errors – May provide adaptative self-care practices via text messaging	– Tied to a specific device brand or model – Controversies on accuracy of BP readings – Lack of transparency and evaluation of the algorithms – Uncertainty of privacy issues and security of data storage
Cuffless measurement through the phone	– No need for devices other than the smartphone – Always available	– Lack of standardization – Low accuracy, no validation for app-related tools

Adapted from Parati et al. [34] by permission

Apps that turn the smartphone into a BP measurement device (cuffless measurement) without the need for ad hoc external devices have also been developed based on measurement principles such as pulse transit time assessment or even without the need for any other device than the smartphone, by applying the subject's finger to the phone camera. Although their extreme ease of use in any circumstance and free availability make them particularly attractive to smartphone users, a major limitation of these apps is the limited evidence from validation studies supporting their accuracy. A recent study evaluating one of these apps indeed indicated that this approach may be highly inaccurate, underestimating higher BP and overestimating lower BP values (mean, SD of the absolute values of the difference between the app and standard were 12.4, 10.5 mmHg for SBP and 10.1, 8.1 mmHg for DBP), thus strongly supporting the need of proper validation of the BP data provided by apps of this kind [16]. The low sensitivity for hypertensive measurements means that approximately four-fifths (77.5%) of individuals with hypertensive BP levels will be falsely reassured that their BP is in the non-hypertensive range. These results have raised awareness on the need to reinforce partnership of app developers, distributors, and regulatory bodies to set and follow standards for safe, validated mHealth technologies.

11.4 BPT: Effects on BP Levels and on Achievement of BP Control

11.4.1 Conventional BPT Systems

Over the last decade, a number of randomized controlled trials as well as their meta-analysis have provided evidence that addition of home BPT is effective in improving adherence and compliance to antihypertensive treatment, achievement of hypertension control, and related medical and economic outcomes in hypertensive patients [4, 12–14, 17–20], especially in those with treatment-resistant hypertension due to poor compliance with multiple drug prescriptions [21] (Fig. 11.2).

In one of the largest meta-analysis of randomized controlled studies including a total of 23 studies ($n = 7,037$ hypertensive patients) regular implementation of BPT at home during a 6-month follow-up period, was associated with significantly greater reductions in both office [average and 95% confidence interval: 4.7 (6.2, 3.2) mmHg for SBP and 2.5 (3.3, 1.6) mmHg for DBP; p<0.001 for both] and 24-hour ambulatory BP [3.5 (5.3, 1.6 mmHg for SBP with p<0.001 and 1.4 (2.9, 0.0) mmHg for DBP with $p = 0.051$], and with a significantly higher chance of achieving office BP normalization [relative risk and 95% confidence interval: 1.16 (1.04, 1.29), $p = 0.007$] as compared to usual care (based on periodic BP measurements and visits at the doctor's office, with no remote BP monitoring) [18]. The improvements in achievement of BP control rates obtained with the BPT intervention resulted in a significantly larger prescription of antihypertensive medications [0.40 (0.17, 0.62), p<0.001], but a similar rate of office consultations. Healthcare costs were significantly (p<0.0001) larger in the BPT group [+662.92 (+540.81, +785.04) euros per

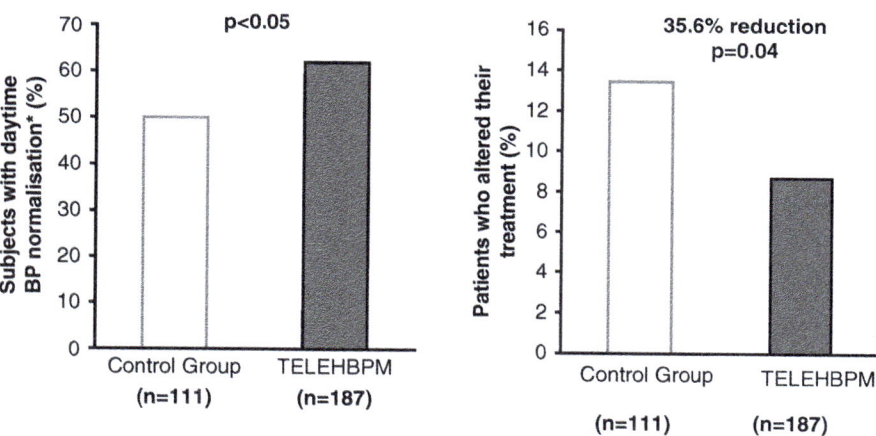

Fig. 11.2 Percentage of patients with daytime ambulatory BP normalization (systolic BP <130 mmHg and diastolic BP <80 mmHg). In this study, hypertensive patients were randomized to be conventionally managed based on office BP measurement (withe bars, $n = 111$) or to be managed based on teletransmission of home BP values (gray bars: $n = 187$). Modified from Parati, et al. [4] by permission

patient], but were similar to those sustained by the patients in the usual care group when costs of the technology were removed and only medical costs were considered [−12.4 (−930.52, +906.23) euros, $p = 0.767$]. More recently, a larger meta-analysis of 46 randomized controlled trials including 13,875 hypertensive patients, further provided evidence on the superiority of BPT in improving achievement of BP control versus usual care [22]. Further relevant evidence on the usefulness of home BPT was recently provided by the TASMINH4 study [5]. This large randomized controlled trial ($n = 1182$) comparatively evaluated the efficacy of self BP monitoring (self-monitoring group, $n = 395$), to self-monitoring blood pressure with telemonitoring (telemonitoring group, $n = 393$), or to usual care (clinic blood pressure; usual care group, n=394) in patients with poorly controlled blood pressure levels. After a 12-month follow-up period, SBP was lower in both intervention groups compared with usual care (self-monitoring, 137·0 [SD 16·7] mm Hg and telemonitoring, 136·0 [16·1] mmHg vs. usual care, 140·4 [16·5]; adjusted mean differences vs. usual care: self-monitoring alone, −3·5 mmHg [95% CI −5·8 to −1·2]; telemonitoring, −4·7 mm Hg [−7·0 to −2·4]). No difference between the self-monitoring and telemonitoring groups was recorded (adjusted mean difference −1·2 mm Hg [95% CI −3·5 to 1·2]), although BP reductions seemed to be quicker in the telemonitoring group.. This study thus showed evidence that self-monitoring, with or without telemonitoring, when used by general practitioners to titrate antihypertensive medication in individuals with poorly controlled blood pressure, leads to significantly lower BP than titration guided by clinic readings [5].

Of note, in most studies a high degree of acceptance of technologies by patients and physicians and a high degree of adherence to telemonitoring programs have been documented [12, 14].

An important aspect of any BPT strategy, is the active participation of health personnel in order to guide patients during BP measurement at home as well as to take decisions regarding therapy [1, 23]. Evidence in this regard was provided by a recent meta-analysis of randomized trials comparing self-monitoring to no-self-monitoring in hypertensive patients by showing that home BPT in conjunction with co-interventions (i.e., medication titration by a case manager, education or lifestyle counselling) may induce significant larger and persistent (up to 12 months) BP reductions than compared to self BP monitoring alone [1] (see Fig. 11.2). Overall, self-monitoring was associated with reduced clinic SBP compared to usual care at 12 months (−3.2 mmHg, [95% CI −4.9, −1.6 mmHg]). However, this effect was strongly influenced by the intensity of co-intervention ranging from no effect with self-monitoring alone (−1.0 mmHg [−3.3, 1.2]), to a 6.1 mmHg (−9.0, −3.2) reduction when monitoring was combined with intensive support [1]. The effectiveness of self-monitoring of BP levels to improve achievement of BP control was shown to be largely dependent on the degree of involvement and participation of health personnel [1] (see Fig. 11.3).

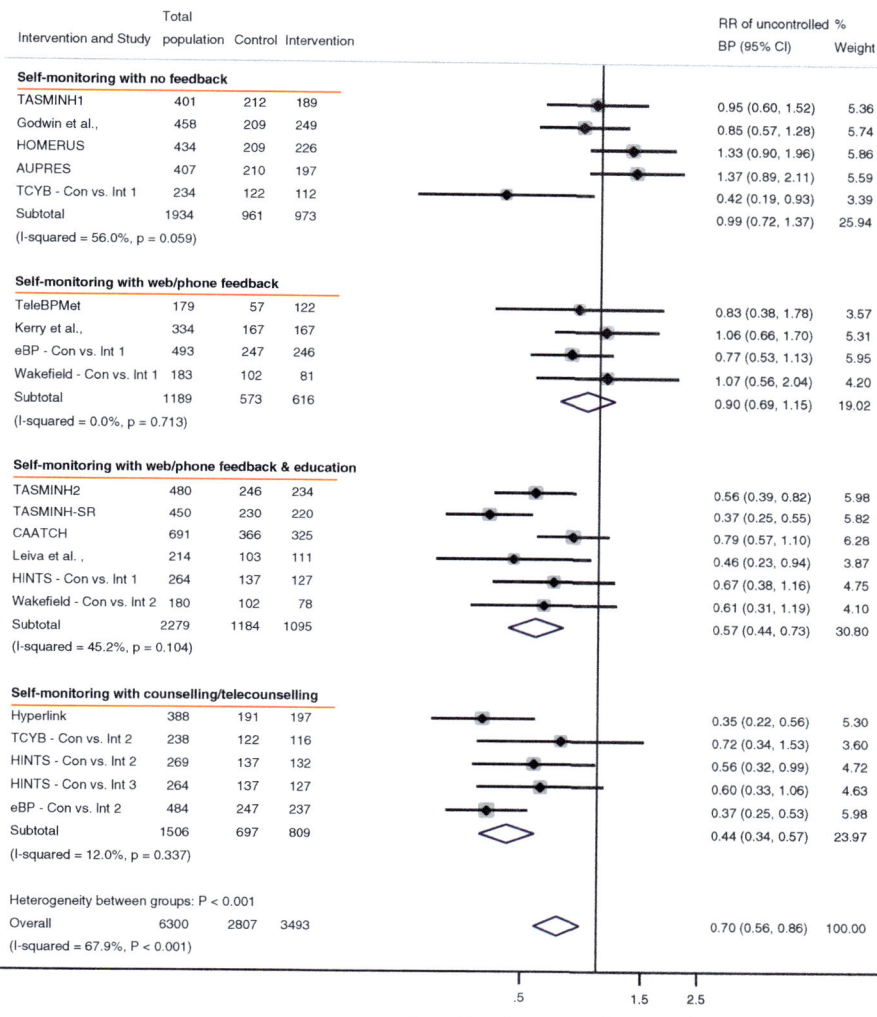

Intervention and Study	Total population	Control	Intervention	RR of uncontrolled % BP (95% CI)	Weight
Self-monitoring with no feedback					
TASMINH1	401	212	189	0.95 (0.60, 1.52)	5.36
Godwin et al.,	458	209	249	0.85 (0.57, 1.28)	5.74
HOMERUS	434	209	226	1.33 (0.90, 1.96)	5.86
AUPRES	407	210	197	1.37 (0.89, 2.11)	5.59
TCYB - Con vs. Int 1	234	122	112	0.42 (0.19, 0.93)	3.39
Subtotal	1934	961	973	0.99 (0.72, 1.37)	25.94
(I-squared = 56.0%, p = 0.059)					
Self-monitoring with web/phone feedback					
TeleBPMet	179	57	122	0.83 (0.38, 1.78)	3.57
Kerry et al.,	334	167	167	1.06 (0.66, 1.70)	5.31
eBP - Con vs. Int 1	493	247	246	0.77 (0.53, 1.13)	5.95
Wakefield - Con vs. Int 1	183	102	81	1.07 (0.56, 2.04)	4.20
Subtotal	1189	573	616	0.90 (0.69, 1.15)	19.02
(I-squared = 0.0%, p = 0.713)					
Self-monitoring with web/phone feedback & education					
TASMINH2	480	246	234	0.56 (0.39, 0.82)	5.98
TASMINH-SR	450	230	220	0.37 (0.25, 0.55)	5.82
CAATCH	691	366	325	0.79 (0.57, 1.10)	6.28
Leiva et al.,	214	103	111	0.46 (0.23, 0.94)	3.87
HINTS - Con vs. Int 1	264	137	127	0.67 (0.38, 1.16)	4.75
Wakefield - Con vs. Int 2	180	102	78	0.61 (0.31, 1.19)	4.10
Subtotal	2279	1184	1095	0.57 (0.44, 0.73)	30.80
(I-squared = 45.2%, p = 0.104)					
Self-monitoring with counselling/telecounselling					
Hyperlink	388	191	197	0.35 (0.22, 0.56)	5.30
TCYB - Con vs. Int 2	238	122	116	0.72 (0.34, 1.53)	3.60
HINTS - Con vs. Int 2	269	137	132	0.56 (0.32, 0.99)	4.72
HINTS - Con vs. Int 3	264	137	127	0.60 (0.33, 1.06)	4.63
eBP - Con vs. Int 2	484	247	237	0.37 (0.25, 0.53)	5.98
Subtotal	1506	697	809	0.44 (0.34, 0.57)	23.97
(I-squared = 12.0%, p = 0.337)					
Heterogeneity between groups: P < 0.001					
Overall	6300	2807	3493	0.70 (0.56, 0.86)	100.00
(I-squared = 67.9%, P < 0.001)					

.5   1.5   2.5

Favours intervention   Favours control

NOTE: Weights are from Random-effects; DerSimonian-Laird estimator

Fig. 11.3 Impact of self-monitoring of BP on the RR of uncontrolled BP at 12 months according to level of co-intervention support (15 studies). Best results were obtained when self-BP monitoring was coupled with web/phone feedback and education or with counselling/telecounselling. Adapted from Tucker et al. [1] by permission. RR of uncontrolled BP adjusted for age, sex, baseline clinic BP, and history of diabetes. The trials are grouped into the four levels of intervention, and *I2* and *P* values are shown for each level of intervention and for the overall analysis. *BP* blood pressure, *RR* relative risk

11.4.2 m-Health BPT Systems

The benefits of BPT based on m-health interventions have also been tested by some clinical trials showing them useful for the management of BP levels and other cardiovascular risk factors (i.e., smoking, blood glucose, lipids, control of body weight) [24–26] being particularly promising for the management of chronic diseases [27] and in conditions characterized by an elevated cardiovascular risk (i.e., for the management of diabetes mellitus patients). In the particular case of hypertension management, preliminary evidence, mostly from small studies, has indicated m-health technologies to be of value to improve achievement of BP control rates and other BP-related outcomes while reducing healthcare costs [6, 20, 28]. In a recent scientific statement of the American Heart Association about the use of mHealth apps for cardiovascular prevention [29] a specific section was dedicated to address the effectiveness of strategies based on mobile apps in achievement of BP control. In the most representative trials that compared mHealth-based BPT strategies versus usual care (consisting of standard visits in the office of a physician), a net reduction in systolic BP of 2.1–8.3 mmHg was detected in favor of the former approach. It should be mentioned, however, that in the vast majority of studies considered for this report, the follow-up was short (less than 12 months, with most of the studies lasting less than 6 months), with no data on mid- to long-term outcomes, which prevented investigators from reliably evaluating adherence to management strategies. Additionally, only three studies used an intention-to-treat approach for data analysis which might have lead to overestimation of the effectiveness of the investigated tools, limiting the applicability of results to real life. Overall, this report highlighted the need for blinded, prospective randomized clinical trials addressing the role of mHealth strategies for BPT, focusing on hard outcomes over longer follow-up times. Evidence in this regard will be provided by the ongoing ESH CARE App project, a joint initiative between the Italian Society of Hypertension and the ESH/ESC aimed at developing and evaluating a new app for BP management. The ESH CARE app allows the user to collect his/her BP values, along with information on ongoing drug therapy (with the possibility to set reminders for pill intake on the phone). It also allows to send the stored BP and heart rate values into a dedicated website, where they are saved in an encrypted end-to-end form. These data may then be managed, organized, and analyzed by a dedicated patient's management system ("Misuriamo" platform), allowing physicians in charge to schematically evaluate BP control, cardiovascular risk level, and drug intake and to more precisely titrate drug prescription, with the consequent possibility to implement an accurate and continuous supervision of patients progress and achieved cardiovascular protection. Preliminary data on the effects of the combined use of the mobile app and the online platform "Misuriamo" (the so-called POST, "Patient Optimal Strategy of Treatment") was tested in a pilot study in Northern Italy [6]. Overall, nine general practitioners randomized 690 consecutive uncontrolled hypertensive patients to either usual care or to the POST strategy. After 6 months of follow-up, achievement of office BP control (i.e., <140/90 mmHg) was significantly higher in the POST group (72.3%) compared to the control group (40.0%). Remarkably, achievement of

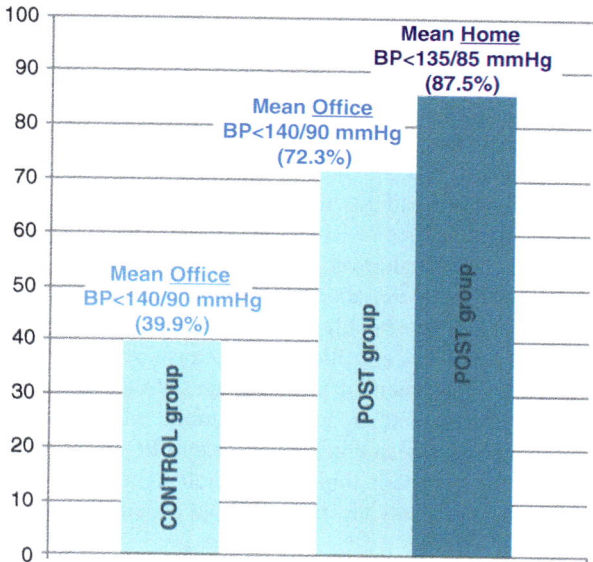

Fig. 11.4 Achievement of office and home BP control in the "Patient Optimal Strategy of Treatment" (POST group) versus control group after 6 months of follow-up in the ESH CARE App project. Data from Albini et al. [6]

Home BP control (i.e., daytime home BP <135/85 mmHg, average of 6 days) in the in the POST group was significantly more frequent than that in office BP levels (87.5% versus 72.3%, respectively), thus strongly supporting the favorable impact of home BPT based on a mHealth strategy for hypertension management (see Fig. 11.4).

Upcoming studies in different countries are being planned to further evaluate the impact on hypertension control by a management strategy based on the ESH CARE app associated to the online platform (the so-called POST strategy), by focusing not only on the possibility of a better control of BP levels over 24 h, but also on the reduction/prevention of organ damage in high-risk hypertensive patients uncontrolled by drug therapy administered according to usual care, and to evaluate whether the POST strategy grants a reduction in cardiovascular mortality and morbidity in hypertensive uncontrolled patients, thus addressing the need of large randomized controlled trials with a long follow-up time.

11.5 Advantages and Limitations of BPT

11.5.1 Conventional BPT

As mentioned above, a major advantage of conventional BPT solutions based on eHealth strategies is the possibility to empower hypertensive patients (patient-centered care) by building feelings of control and support for chronic disease self-management [30]. BPT facilitates patients to communicate with their doctors, without the need to travel long distances, which translates into a decreased transportation burden and time savings [31]. In due course, physicians and health-care professionals may reach patients beyond their office, track their health status, and quickly and easily communicate with them. This represents an important advantage for the management of a chronic disease such as hypertension by allowing a closer long-term follow-up of treated hypertensive patients. In case of poor BP control or in the presence of acute symptoms or sudden BP rises, physicians may indeed easily indicate patients to alter their health behaviors or modify antihypertensive medication between visits, avoiding the need to wait months between visits for adjustments. In addition, several BPT systems allow sending automatic reminders to patients indicating the time of BP measurement and/or of medication intake, and may also alert the health provider about new changes in a patient's health that may manifest with uncontrolled BP. Because of these unique characteristics, BPT systems have the potential to overcome not only physicians' inertia but also patients' low compliance/adherence to treatment, which ultimately translates into improvements in hypertension control rates and BP-related cardiovascular complications.

Despite all these important benefits, implementation of BPT solutions in the daily practice may be difficult due to cultural, structural, or financial barriers (Table 11.3) [32].

Poor informatics skill levels of healthcare professionals and patients, lack of adequate knowledge of BP measurement and hypertension guidelines by doctors, all represent major cultural barriers to the routine use of BPT. The incomplete evidence on the clinical efficacy and economic benefit of BPT provided so far by randomized studies, technological barriers, high costs of devices, heterogeneity of solutions and technologies, lack of infrastructures and standards, all hinder the dissemination of telehealth strategies. Regarding the duration of the studies, most current evidence on BPT is based on studies of relatively short duration

Table 11.3 Current barriers to the adoption of blood pressure telemonitoring

Cultural barriers
- Poor informatics literacy of healthcare workforces and patients
- Lack of adequate knowledge and proper implementation of BP monitoring guidelines by doctors
- Unawareness of the importance of cardiovascular risk factors detection and control among people
- Need of more robust evidence on the benefit of BPT, focusing studies on BPT solutions provided with co-intervention

Structural barriers
- Lack of adequate infrastructures (mobile network, Internet, connected homes)
- Need for simple and user-friendly devices, possibly integrated in mobile phones, tablets or home appliances
- Need to ensure data integrity, security and privacy

Financial barriers
- Need of cost-effective systems (full demonstration lacking)
- Need for cheap and integrated devices
- Lack of reimbursement models

Adapted by permission from Parati et al. [14] by permission
BP blood pressure, *BPT* blood pressure telemonitoring

(<12 months) and in the few studies looking at longer-term outcomes, no evidence of better or sustained effect could be provided. Additionally, no definition of the optimal BPT-based healthcare delivery model could be derived from the studies performed so far, due to the heterogeneity of interventions, technologies and study designs.

11.5.2 mHealth-Based BPT Systems

Mobile phones, which had been traditionally used for communications between patients and doctors only (i.e., through phone calls or SMS) [33], have not only presented a widespread use in recent years but have also expanded their applications giving new possibilities for improving BPT systems [34]. Mobile phones may indeed provide wireless diagnostic and clinical decision support tools to healthcare providers for monitoring health status or improving health outcomes, overcoming many of the technical and financial difficulties (installation and maintenance costs) of conventional BPT systems. Smartphone apps can empower patients with accurate medical information (i.e., educational sections), provide tools to promote self-monitoring and self-management, tracking services (body weight, physical activity), and encourage greater participation in medical decision making by tools that improve adherence to treatment (through reminders and tracking of drug intake) [35]. Mobile phones may thus represent an excellent tool to improve hypertension management in a population basis, i.e., by allowing billions of people to regularly check their BP status and to turn a mobile appliance into an important tool for improving BP control and cardiovascular risk prevention.

Although it is unquestionable that the increasing use of m-health technologies due to the large availability of user-friendly smartphones will circumvent the technical challenge of BPT and provide more flexible and cheap platforms to enhance patient care, it should be mentioned, however that the development and diffusion of these solutions in most cases, has not been accompanied by validation studies (i.e., in order to evaluate their accuracy in measuring biological variables) and standardization of protocols for data transmission and use. Indeed, while a large number of apps dedicated to hypertension management and, in general, related to health issues can be found on web stores, only very few of them can be considered accurate and safe for clinical use.

A critical meta-analysis of 107 mobile health applications designed for the management of hypertension found that only 2.8% of the apps were developed by healthcare professional agencies, none provided any documentation of validation against a gold standard in patients with hypertension, and none formally obtained approval for use as a measuring device by the US Food and Drug Administration or EC [35]. The same meta-analysis also showed that while many apps are positioned in the market and in the online stores based on their popularity rankings (i.e., number of downloads by users) there are still no guidelines nor critical and standardized methods for validating their quality, accuracy, efficacy and safety based on scientific criteria, in order to recommend their use for clinical purposes [35]. Because of all these critical issues, the great opportunity for the improvement of individual and public health carried by mHealth solutions might paradoxically turn into a possible risk for users. Assessing mobile apps is a challenge, we need adapted guidelines and expert and end user evaluation [36].

Another important limitation of studies addressing the value of mhealth systems for BPT is the extremely high level of heterogeneity among them, i.e., almost every smartphone producer has already developed its own healthcare-related app, along with accessories like smartbands and smartwatches, for detection of BP levels and related hemodynamic variables (i.e., heart rate, heart rate variability, physical activity, sleep quality). Lack of standardization in this field does indeed represent a factor that could hamper the possibility of summarizing data on impact on outcome and of drawing general assumptions and reducing the strength of the evidence provided. Future research needs to explore the specific outcomes of BPT interventions to determine their relative value. It should also determine which BPT provision model best applies to daily clinical practice and gives the maximum benefit. Such studies should particularly be focused on high-risk hypertensive patients, for whom an optimal BP control is particularly difficult to attain, also evaluating whether the benefit of BPT intervention is sustained in the long term.

Although there is still limited evidence on the use of mHealth technologies in hypertension management, a list of potential benefits and drawbacks in hypertension management is reported in Table 11.4.

Table 11.4 Potential benefits and limitations of m-health for hypertension management

Medical benefits
- Enhanced communication between patient and physician (improvement of patient's adherence to treatment and physician's inertia)
- Increased patient's education on its condition
- Patient empowering by promotion of self-managing and encouraging greater participation in medical decision making
- Improved control of risk factors and health status, particularly for patients with chronic conditions (but few evidence and only on the short term)

Practical benefits
- Remote monitoring of patients difficult to reach or needing strict surveillance
- Low network maintenance
- Phones are always on, computers are not
- Carrying a phone or a tablet is part of a modern lifestyle
- Using a small portable multi-communication computing device is convenient, economical, practical and personal

Drawbacks
- No proper regulation, standardization and validation of the development process of m-Health technologies
- Absence of a critical and standardized method for the quality evaluation of m-apps
- These tools are not yet considered medical devices (most are enlisted in the "fitness" or "wellness" category)
- Few of m-apps for hypertension can be regarded as accurate and safe for clinical use
- Potential privacy and security issues (sensitive data)

Adapted by permission from Parati et al. [14]

11.6 Conclusions

Increasing evidence has indicated a substantial contribution of telemedicine and Information Technology to Hypertension management. When properly implemented on a regular basis, the combined use of devices that allow patients to self-measure BP at home, transmit the reading to their doctors, and get a feedback could induce an increased compliance through education and involvement of the patients in the management of their own health, plus improving doctor-patients relationship. Current evidence suggests that conventional BPT systems based on eHealth technologies not only have the potential to improve achievement of hypertension control rates, but also to enhance cardiovascular protection by preventing the cardiovascular consequences associated with elevated BP levels. This is of particular value in patients needing a tighter BP control (e.g., at high cardiovascular risk or with comorbidities) or requiring monitoring of multiple vital signs. BPT is in general well accepted by patients and may help to reduce the frequency of face-to-face consultations, and to avoid unnecessary clinic access. In the last instance, such an approach would translate in increased health and reduced restrain healthcare expenditure (i.e., human and technical costs). The increasing number of available mobile apps related to hypertension management and their usage by smartphone owners has led to the recent introduction of BPT solutions based on m-health technology. Although preliminary data from small studies have suggested the efficacy of these technologies to increase patients' compliance and adherence to antihypertensive treatment, thus improving rates of BP control, evidence is still needed from validation studies evaluating their accuracy as well as from population-based outcome studies showing whether implementing these technologies may result in benefits for the long-term management of hypertension and to improve cardiovascular protection.

Acknowledgment *Disclosure*: SO is scientific consultant of Biotechmed Ltd. provider of telemedicine services.

References

1. Tucker KL, Sheppard JP, Stevens R, Bosworth HB, Bove A, Bray EP, et al. Self-monitoring of blood pressure in hypertension: a systematic review and individual patient data meta-analysis. PLoS Med. 2017;14(9):e1002389.
2. Whelton PK, Carey RM, Aronow WS, Casey DE Jr, Collins KJ, Dennison Himmelfarb C, et al. 2017 ACC/AHA/AAPA/ABC/ACPM/AGS/APhA/ASH/ASPC/NMA/PCNA guideline for the prevention, detection, evaluation, and management of high blood pressure in adults: a report of the American College of Cardiology/American Heart Association task force on clinical practice guidelines. Hypertension. 2018;71(6):e13–e115.
3. Williams B, Mancia G, Spiering W, Agabiti Rosei E, Azizi M, Burnier M, et al. 2018 Practice Guidelines for the management of arterial hypertension of the European Society of Hypertension and the European Society of Cardiology: ESH/ESC Task Force for the Management of Arterial Hypertension. J Hypertens. 2018;36(12):2284–309.
4. Parati G, Omboni S, Albini F, Piantoni L, Giuliano A, Revera M, et al. Home blood pressure telemonitoring improves hypertension control in general practice. The TeleBPCare study. J Hypertens. 2009;27(1):198–203.

5. McManus RJ, Mant J, Franssen M, Nickless A, Schwartz C, Hodgkinson J, et al. Efficacy of self-monitored blood pressure, with or without telemonitoring, for titration of antihypertensive medication (TASMINH4): an unmasked randomised controlled trial. Lancet. 2018;391(10124):949–59.
6. Albini F, Xiaoqiu L, Torlasco C, Soranna D, Faini A, Ciminaghi R, et al. An ICT and mobile health integrated approach to optimize patients' education on hypertension and its management by physicians: the patients optimal strategy of treatment(POST) pilot study. Conf Proc IEEE Eng Med Biol Soc. 2016;2016:517–20.
7. Sood S, Mbarika V, Jugoo S, Dookhy R, Doarn CR, Prakash N, et al. What is telemedicine? A collection of 104 peer-reviewed perspectives and theoretical underpinnings. Telemed J E Health. 2007;13(5):573–90.
8. TR. E. The eHealth Landscape: A Terrain Map of Emerging Information and Communication Technologies in Health and Health Care;2001.
9. Silva BM, Rodrigues JJ, de la Torre Diez I, Lopez-Coronado M, Saleem K. Mobile-health: a review of current state in 2015. J Biomed Inform. 2015;56:265–72.
10. Akter S, D'Ambra J. P. R. Trustworthiness in mHealth information services: an assessment of a hierarchical model with mediating and moderating effects using partial least squares (PLS). J Am Soc Inf Sci Technol. 2011;62:100–16.
11. Baig MM, GholamHosseini H, Connolly MJ. Mobile healthcare applications: system design review, critical issues and challenges. Australas Phys Eng Sci Med. 2015;38(1):23–38.
12. Omboni S, Ferrari R. The role of telemedicine in hypertension management: focus on blood pressure telemonitoring. Curr Hypertens Rep. 2015;17(4):535.
13. Parati G, Omboni S. Role of home blood pressure telemonitoring in hypertension management: an update. Blood Press Monit. 2010;15(6):285–95.
14. Parati G, Dolan E, McManus RJ, Omboni S. Home blood pressure telemonitoring in the 21st century. J Clin Hypertens (Greenwich). 2018;20(7):1128–32.
15. Grim CE. Home blood pressure devices for the iPhone do not get the same readings on the same person. J Am Soc Hypertens. 2014;8:e54–5.
16. Plante TB, Urrea B, MacFarlane ZT, Blumenthal RS, Miller ER 3rd, Appel LJ, et al. Validation of the instant blood pressure smartphone app. JAMA Intern Med. 2016;176(5):700–2.
17. Collaborators GBDRF, Forouzanfar MH, Alexander L, Anderson HR, Bachman VF, Biryukov S, et al. Global, regional, and national comparative risk assessment of 79 behavioural, environmental and occupational, and metabolic risks or clusters of risks in 188 countries, 1990–2013: a systematic analysis for the Global Burden of Disease Study 2013. Lancet. 2015;386(10010):2287–323.
18. Omboni S, Gazzola T, Carabelli G, Parati G. Clinical usefulness and cost effectiveness of home blood pressure telemonitoring: meta-analysis of randomized controlled studies. J Hypertens. 2013;31(3):455–67;discussion 467-8.
19. Omboni S, Guarda A. Impact of home blood pressure telemonitoring and blood pressure control: a meta-analysis of randomized controlled studies. Am J Hypertens. 2011;24(9):989–98.
20. Omboni S, Caserini M, Coronetti C. Telemedicine and M-health in hypertension management: technologies, applications and clinical evidence. High Blood Press Cardiovasc Prev. 2016;23(3):187–96.
21. Ogedegbe G, Schoenthaler A. A systematic review of the effects of home blood pressure monitoring on medication adherence. J Clin Hypertens (Greenwich). 2006;8(3):174–80.
22. Duan Y, Xie Z, Dong F, Wu Z, Lin Z, Sun N, et al. Effectiveness of home blood pressure telemonitoring: a systematic review and meta-analysis of randomised controlled studies. J Hum Hypertens. 2017;31(7):427–37.
23. Uhlig K, Patel K, Ip S, Kitsios GD, Balk EM. Self-measured blood pressure monitoring in the management of hypertension: a systematic review and meta-analysis. Ann Intern Med. 2013;159(3):185–94.
24. Quinn CC, Clough SS, Minor JM, Lender D, Okafor MC, Gruber-Baldini A. WellDoc mobile diabetes management randomized controlled trial: change in clinical and behavioral outcomes and patient and physician satisfaction. Diabetes Technol Ther. 2008;10(3):160–8.

25. Quinn CC, Shardell MD, Terrin ML, Barr EA, Ballew SH, Gruber-Baldini AL. Cluster-randomized trial of a mobile phone personalized behavioral intervention for blood glucose control. Diabetes Care. 2011;34(9):1934–42.
26. Liang X, Wang Q, Yang X, Cao J, Chen J, Mo X, et al. Effect of mobile phone intervention for diabetes on glycaemic control: a meta-analysis. Diabet Med. 2011;28(4):455–63.
27. Goldberg EM, Levy PD. New approaches to evaluating and monitoring blood pressure. Curr Hypertens Rep. 2016;18(6):49.
28. Purcell R, McInnes S, Halcomb EJ. Telemonitoring can assist in managing cardiovascular disease in primary care: a systematic review of systematic reviews. BMC Fam Pract. 2014;15:43.
29. Burke LE, Ma J, Azar KM, Bennett GG, Peterson ED, Zheng Y, et al. Current science on consumer use of mobile health for cardiovascular disease prevention: a scientific statement from the American Heart Association. Circulation. 2015;132(12):1157–213.
30. Cottrell E, McMillan K, Chambers R. A cross-sectional survey and service evaluation of simple telehealth in primary care: what do patients think? BMJ Open. 2012;2(6)
31. Friedman RH. Automated telephone conversations to assess health behavior and deliver behavioral interventions. J Med Syst. 1998;22(2):95–102.
32. Wood PW, Boulanger P, Padwal RS. Home blood pressure telemonitoring: rationale for use, required elements, and barriers to implementation in Canada. Can J Cardiol. 2017;33(5):619–25.
33. de Jongh T, Gurol-Urganci I, Vodopivec-Jamsek V, Car J, Atun R. Mobile phone messaging for facilitating self-management of long-term illnesses. Cochrane Database Syst Rev. 2012;12:CD007459.
34. Parati G, Torlasco C, Omboni S, Pellegrini D. Smartphone applications for hypertension management: a potential game-changer that needs more control. Curr Hypertens Rep. 2017;19(6):48.
35. Kumar N, Khunger M, Gupta A, Garg N. A content analysis of smartphone-based applications for hypertension management. J Am Soc Hypertens. 2015;9(2):130–6.
36. Ranasinghe M, Cabrera A, Postel-Vinay N, Boyer C. Transparency and quality of health apps: the HON approach. Stud Health Technol Inform. 2018;247:656–60.

Nocturnal Home Blood Pressure Monitoring

12

George S. Stergiou, Emmanuel Andreadis, Kei Asayama,
Kazuomi Kario, Anastasios Kollias, Takayoshi Ohkubo,
Gianfranco Parati, Michael A. Weber, and Yutaka Imai

G. S. Stergiou (✉)
Hypertension Center STRIDE-7, National and Kapodistrian University of Athens, School of
Medicine, Third Department of Medicine, Sotiria Hospital, Athens, Greece
e-mail: gstergi@med.uoa.gr

A. Kollias
Hypertension Center STRIDE-7, National and Kapodistrian University of Athens, School of
Medicine, Third Department of Medicine, Sotiria Hospital, Athens, Greece

E. Andreadis
Chairman of Fourth Internal Medicine Department, Head of Hypertension and Cardiovascular
Disease Prevention Center, Evangelismos General Hospital, Athens, Greece

K. Asayama
Department of Hygiene and Public Health, Teikyo University School of Medicine,
Tokyo, Japan

Tohoku Institute for Management of Blood Pressure, Sendai, Japan

Studies Coordinating Centre, Research Unit Hypertension and Cardiovascular Epidemiology,
KU Leuven Department of Cardiovascular Sciences, University of Leuven, Leuven, Belgium
e-mail: kei@asayama.org

T. Ohkubo
Department of Hygiene and Public Health, Teikyo University School of Medicine,
Tokyo, Japan

Tohoku Institute for Management of Blood Pressure, Sendai, Japan
e-mail: tohkubo@med.teikyo-u.ac.jp

K. Kario
Division of Cardiovascular Medicine, Department of Medicine, Jichi Medical University
School of Medicine (JMU), Tochigi, Japan
e-mail: kkario@jichi.ac.jp

G. Parati
Department of Medicine and Surgery, University of Milano-Bicocca, Milan, Italy

Istituto Auxologico Italiano, IRCCS, Department of Cardiovascular, Neural and Metabolic
Sciences, Milan, Italy
e-mail: gianfranco.parati@unimib.it

G. S. Stergiou et al. (eds.), *Home Blood Pressure Monitoring*,
Updates in Hypertension and Cardiovascular Protection,
https://doi.org/10.1007/978-3-030-23065-4_12

M. A. Weber
Division of Cardiovascular Medicine, State University of New York, Downstate Medical
Center, New York, NY, USA

Y. Imai
Tohoku Institute for Management of Blood Pressure, Sendai, Japan
e-mail: yutaka.imai.d6@tohoku.ac.jp

12.1   Introduction

A unique feature of 24-h ambulatory blood pressure monitoring (ABPM) is its ability
to evaluate blood pressure (BP) during nighttime sleep [1]. This is an important
advantage of the method because nighttime ABPM has been shown to have the strongest prognostic value compared to all the other BP measurement methods [1–3]. The
modern technology of devices for self-home BP monitoring (HBPM) has provided
low-cost devices which are programmed to allow automated BP measurements during nighttime [4]. In 2001 Yutaka Imai and coworkers published the first study presenting a novel HBPM device (Omron HEM-747 IC-N) which was able to take
automated BP measurement during nighttime sleep [5]. In the last 17 years several
studies assessed the feasibility and applicability of nocturnal HBPM and compared
with ABPM in terms of asleep BP values and their association with indices of preclinical organ damage. An international consensus presenting the available evidence
[5–16] and the advantages of nocturnal HBPM was recently published (Table 12.1)
[4]. The chapter summarizes the published evidence on nocturnal HBPM aiming to
define its potential in the evaluation of hypertensive patients in clinical practice.

12.2   Nocturnal Home Versus Ambulatory Blood Pressure

Nocturnal HBPM has been investigated as an alternative to ABPM, which is the
reference method for the evaluation of nighttime sleep BP and the detection of non-
dippers [1]. A cross-sectional study which investigated 81 hypertensive subjects
using 24-h ABPM and HBPM using a device developed to take automated measurements during nighttime sleep (Microlife WatchBP Home N, Microlife AG, Widnau,
Switzerland) showed similar daytime and nighttime BP values and 74% agreement
between the two methods in detecting non-dippers (Fig. 12.1) [9]. This agreement
between HBPM and ABPM is similar to the reproducibility of non-dippers using
repeat ABPM and, therefore, suggests that these methods appear to be interchangeable for diagnosing the non-dipping patter [17, 18]. A recent meta-analysis of 6
studies (3 in Japan, 2 in Greece, 1 in Finland) including 1404 subjects compared
nocturnal HBPM with ABPM and showed pooled difference 1.4/−0.2 mmHg (sys-
tolic/diastolic) and pooled correlation coefficient between them 0.70/0.72 (Fig. 12.2)
[19]. In the same meta-analysis, 2 studies including 212 subjects investigated the
agreement between nocturnal HBPM and ABPM in detecting non-dippers and
showed weighted agreement 77% [19]. These preliminary data suggest that nocturnal HBPM appears to be a reliable alternative to ABPM for the evaluation of asleep
BP and the detection of non-dippers.

Table 12.1 Characteristics of studies investigating nocturnal home blood pressure (with permission from [4])

Author (Year)	Recruitment (country)	No. Participants (% women)	Age, years (SD)	Device Model (Company)	Measurement days (intervals)	Measurements per night	Systolic BP, mmHg	Diastolic BP, mmHg	Sleep quality assessment
Observational									
Chonan (2001) [5]	HT (Japan)	49 (–)	–	HEM-747IC-N (Omron)	10 (1)	1 (2 am)	118.6	72.8	At each post-measurement
Hosohata (2007) [6]	P (Japan)	556 (71)	62 (11)	HEM-747IC-N (Omron)	2 (6)	1 (2 am)	116.8	68.0	At each post-measurement
Ushio (2009) [7]	V (Japan)	40 (30)	25 (5)	HEM-5041 (Omron)	7 (1)	6 (1 h interval)	107.6	59.3	After the measurement completion
Ishikawa (2012) [8]	GP (Japan)	854 (53)	63 (11)	HEM-5001 (Omron)	9 (≥1 per wk)	3 (2, 3, 4 am)	123.0	70.2	None
Stergiou (2012) [9]	HT (Greece)	81 (47)	58 (11)	WatchBPN (microlife)	3 (1)	3 (2, 3, 4 h after going to bed)	114.1	66.4	After the measurement completion
Stergiou (2013) [10]	OSA (Greece)	39 (28)	49 (11)	WatchBPN (microlife)	3 (1)	3 (2, 3, 4 h after going to bed)	115.1	69.3	Polysomnography
Andreadis (2016) [11]	HT (Greece)	131 (42)	52 (12)	WatchBPN (microlife)	3 (1)	3 (2, 3, 4 h after going to bed)	122.4	73.9	None
Lindroos (2016) [12, 13]	P (Finland)	248 (55)	58 (13)	WatchBP home N (microlife)	2 (1)	3 (2, 3, 4 h after going to bed)	113.0	65.2	After the measurement completion
Clinical trial									
Kario (2010) [14]	HT (Japan)	161 (53)	67 (13)	HEM-5001 (Omron)	7 (1)	3 (2, 3, 4 am)	131.6	75.7	None
Kario (2017) [15]	HT (Japan)	411 (45)	63 (12)	HEM-7252G-HP (Omron)	5 (1)	3 (2, 3, 4 am)	128.3	79.3	None
Fujiwara (2018) [16]	HT (Japan)	129 (57)	68 (12)	HEM-7252G-HP (Omron)	3 (during 4 wk)	3 (2, 3, 4 am)	125.1	76.3	None

BP blood pressure, *HT* hypertensive patients, *P* general population, *V* healthy volunteers, *GP* outpatient clinic, *OSA* obstructive sleep apnea, *–* not available, *wk* week. When two or more papers were published from the single study, data from the initial report were extracted

Ambulatory BP
Home BP
AGREEMENT IN DETECTING NON-DIPPERS 74%
mmHg
130
120
110
100
90
80
70
60
Day SBP
Night SBP
Day DBP
Night DBP

Fig. 12.1 Comparison of awake and asleep home and ambulatory blood pressure measurements (with permission from [9])

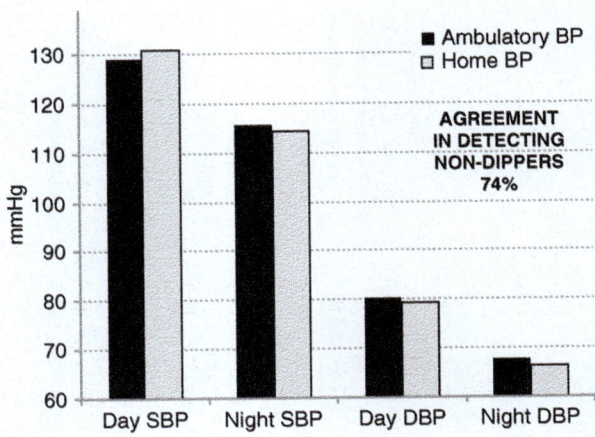

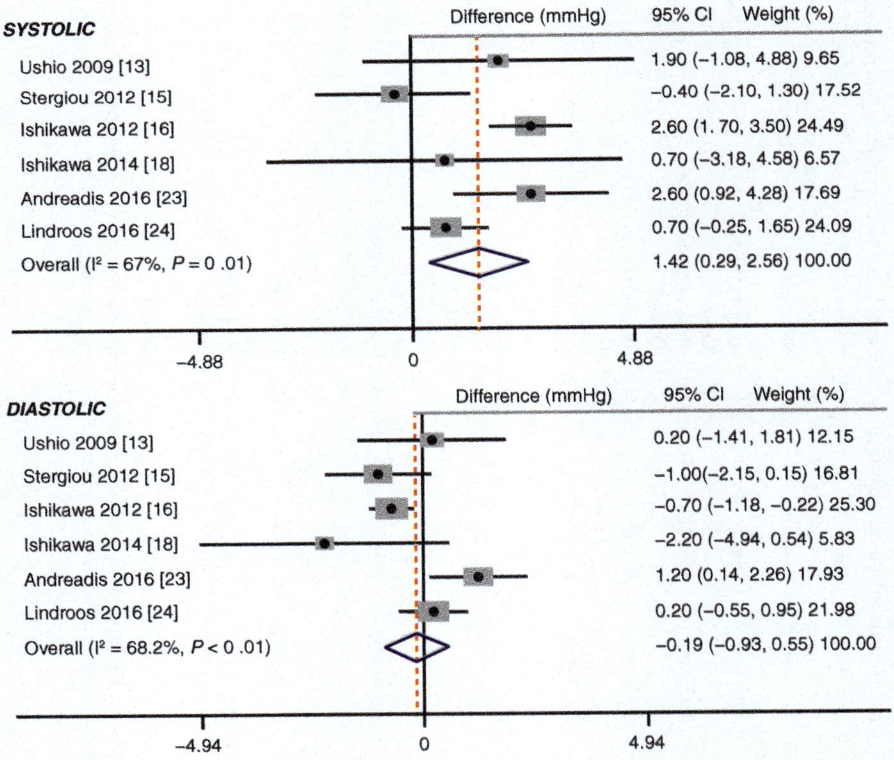

SYSTOLIC
Difference (mmHg)
95% CI Weight (%)
Ushio 2009 [13]
1.90 (−1.08, 4.88) 9.65
Stergiou 2012 [15]
−0.40 (−2.10, 1.30) 17.52
Ishikawa 2012 [16]
2.60 (1. 70, 3.50) 24.49
Ishikawa 2014 [18]
0.70 (−3.18, 4.58) 6.57
Andreadis 2016 [23]
2.60 (0.92, 4.28) 17.69
Lindroos 2016 [24]
0.70 (−0.25, 1.65) 24.09
Overall (I² = 67%, P = 0 .01)
1.42 (0.29, 2.56) 100.00
−4.88
0
4.88
DIASTOLIC
Difference (mmHg)
95% CI Weight (%)
Ushio 2009 [13]
0.20 (−1.41, 1.81) 12.15
Stergiou 2012 [15]
−1.00(−2.15, 0.15) 16.81
Ishikawa 2012 [16]
−0.70 (−1.18, −0.22) 25.30
Ishikawa 2014 [18]
−2.20 (−4.94, 0.54) 5.83
Andreadis 2016 [23]
1.20 (0.14, 2.26) 17.93
Lindroos 2016 [24]
0.20 (−0.55, 0.95) 21.98
Overall (I² = 68.2%, P < 0 .01)
−0.19 (−0.93, 0.55) 100.00
−4.94
0
4.94

Fig. 12.2 Meta-analysis of studies comparing home versus ambulatory nighttime blood pressure (with permission from [19])

12.3 Relationship of Nocturnal Home Blood Pressure with Preclinical Organ Damage

Nocturnal hypertension and the non-dipping BP pattern assessed by 24-h ABPM have been shown to be associated with several indices of preclinical target organ damage as well as with cardiovascular events [1–3, 20]. Three studies conducted in Japan [8], Greece [11], and Finland [12] compared nocturnal HBPM versus ABPM in terms of their association with echocardiographic left ventricular mass index, urine albumin excretion, and carotid intima-media thickness in general population and in subjects with hypertension and/or other cardiovascular risk factors. A meta-analysis of these data showed similar pooled correlation coefficients for left ventricular mass index ($n = 954$; $r = 0.36$ and 0.32, respectively, for nocturnal systolic HBPM versus ABPM), urine albumin excretion ($n = 950$; $r = 0.39$ versus 0.30), and carotid intima-media thickness ($n = 350$; $r = 0.31$ versus 0.35) [19]. Furthermore, Kario et al. showed that the mean sleep BP among 2562 participants of the Japan Morning Surge Home Blood Pressure (J-HOP) study who self-measured their BP during sleep using a validated home monitor was closely associated with the development of preclinical target organ damage, as well as with elevated plasma NT-proBNP, even after controlling for clinic systolic BPs and home morning and evening systolic BPs. Interestingly, 27% of the studied population with well controlled morning home BP was identified as having masked home nocturnal hypertension, which highlights the clinical value of nocturnal HBPM [21]. Moreover, it has been showed that masked uncontrolled nocturnal hypertension further increases cardiovascular risk among hypertensive subjects [22]. In a 41-subject sub-study of the Japan Morning Surge-Target Organ Protection (J-TOP), the decline in nocturnal systolic home BP, but not in ambulatory BP, induced by the antihypertensive drug treatment was associated with regression of left ventricular mass index [23]. These data suggest that nocturnal HBPM is closely associated with indices of preclinical target organ damage, with similar correlation coefficients as those obtained by ABPM, and can predict the antihypertensive treatment-induced regression in left ventricular hypertrophy at least as efficiently as ABPM.

12.4 Optimal Nocturnal Home Blood Pressure Monitoring Schedule

The currently available studies which compared nocturnal HBPM with ABPM have considerable heterogeneity in the schedule applied for nocturnal HBPM, ranging from total of 3–6 readings per night and from 2 or as many nights as possible during 2 weeks [19]. A recent meta-regression analysis did not reveal a significant impact of the number of nighttime HBPM readings obtained across the meta-analyzed studies on the nighttime home minus ambulatory BP difference [19]. A single study in untreated hypertensives investigated the optimal nocturnal HBPM schedule in terms of the number of BP readings per night and the number of nights required [19]. The analysis suggested that a 2-night HBPM schedule (total of 6 readings) appears to be the minimum requirement for a reliable assessment of nighttime HBPM, providing reasonable agreement with nocturnal ABPM values and association with indices of preclinical organ damage (Fig. 12.3). These finding are in line with the current ABPM recommendations for a minimum requirement of 7 readings for the assessment of nighttime ambulatory BP [1].

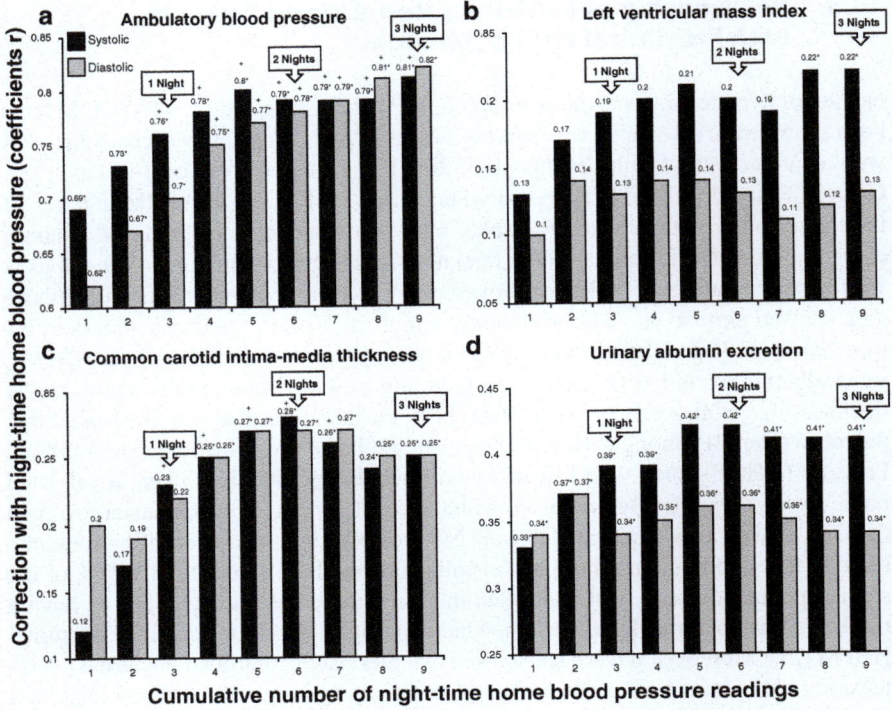

Fig. 12.3 Effect of averaging an increasing number of nighttime home blood pressure readings on its relationship with nighttime ambulatory blood pressure and indices of target organ damage (+, P < 0.05; * P < 0.05 versus first reading) (with permission from [24])

12.5 Further Applications and Development of Nocturnal Home Blood Pressure Monitoring

Obstructive sleep apnea is known to be associated with nocturnal BP elevation and non-dipping profile assessed by ABPM, increasing thereby the cardiovascular risk [1]. A pilot study in 39 subjects referred to a sleep clinic for polysomnography were assessed with conventional office BP measurements and HBPM including automated nighttime sleep measurements (3 readings per night for 3 nights) [24]. The study showed a consistent trend towards stronger correlations of the nighttime diastolic HBPM readings with the apnea severity (apnea-hypopnea index, duration of desaturation, maximum and minimum arterial oxygen saturation) and in multivariate analysis the apnea-hypopnea index was independently associated with nighttime diastolic home BP [10]. A novel home BP monitor has been developed specifically for the evaluation of patients with obstructive sleep apnea, which is able to trigger sleep BP measurement during episodes of hypoxia (reduced oxygen desaturation) [25, 26]. Thus, nocturnal HBPM has the potential to replace ABPM in the investigation of nocturnal BP in patients with sleep apnea and also to evaluate asleep BP in succeeding nights.

Nocturnal HBPM has the advantage to be able to provide long-term monitoring for months, which is not possible with 24-h ABPM. Nocturnal HBPM has been used in a cross-sectional general population study in 4780 subjects in Japan, aiming to assess the seasonal variation in BP levels [27]. Measurements of BP were taken at home for several days during daytime and nighttime using an automated HBPM device and sleeping times were evaluated by actigraphy. The study showed that the nocturnal home BP fall considerably differs in different seasons, with higher prevalence of nighttime rising and non-dipping pattern in summer [27], which is in line with the findings using ABPM [28].

Novel nocturnal home BP telemonitoring devices have been developed based on new communication technology (ICT) systems. Their novelty is that they directly transmit the patient's home BP measurements as they are recorded during nighttime. Recent multicenter randomized controlled trials showed that these devices can be widely used by hypertensive subjects [15, 29]. Moreover, some data suggest that nocturnal HBPM might be an alternative to ABPM for the measurement of nighttime BP, nocturnal BP fall, morning BP surge, and other indices of the BP profile, which affect cardiovascular outcomes. The effects of antihypertensive drug treatment on reducing home morning blood pressure surge has been investigated in an attempt to reduce cardiovascular morbidity and mortality [16].

One issue with both nocturnal HBPM and ABPM is that the inflation of the arm cuff during sleep results in arm compression which may affect the sleep level and thereby the BP level [30–32]. A wrist-cuff HBPM device has been recently developed (Omron HEM6310F-N, Omron Healthcare, Co. Ltd., Kyoto, Japan) which takes measurements with less pump noise and faster inflation [33]. A study in 57 subjects showed lower nocturnal BP and also less sleep disturbance with the wrist than the arm-cuff home monitor (20% of subjects versus 70% with the arm device), which might result in more accurate evaluation of nighttime BP [33].

12.6   Conclusion

Accumulating evidence suggests that the evaluation of BP during nighttime sleep using modern low-cost automated home BP monitors is feasible and provides information which is clinically relevant and similar to that provided by nighttime ABPM. More research is required, particularly with long-term trials, in order to demonstrate the exact role of nocturnal HBPM and verify its role in improving the management of patients with hypertension in clinical practice.

References

1. O'Brien E, Parati G, Stergiou G, Asmar R, Beilin L, Bilo G, et al. European Society of Hypertension position paper on ambulatory blood pressure monitoring. J Hypertens. 2013;31(9):1731–68.

2. Hansen TW, Li Y, Boggia J, Thijs L, Richart T, Staessen JA. Predictive role of the night-time blood pressure. Hypertension. 2011;57:3–10.
3. Fagard RH, Celis H, Thijs L, Staessen JA, Clement DL, De Buyzere ML, et al. Daytime and night-time blood pressure as predictors of death and cause-specific cardiovascular events in hypertension. Hypertension. 2008;51:55–61.
4. Asayama K, Fujiwara T, Hoshide S, Ohkubo T, Kario K, Stergiou GS, et al. Nocturnal blood pressure measured by home devices: evidence and perspective for clinical application. J Hypertens. 2019;37(5):905–16.
5. Chonan K, Kikuya M, Araki T, Fujiwara T, Suzuki M, Michimata M, et al. Device for the self-measurement of blood pressure that can monitor blood pressure during sleep. Blood Press Monit. 2001;6(4):203–5.
6. Hosohata K, Kikuya M, Ohkubo T, Metoki H, Asayama K, Inoue R, et al. Reproducibility of nocturnal blood pressure assessed by self-measurement of blood pressure at home. Hypertens Res. 2007;30:707–12.
7. Ushio H, Ishigami T, Araki N, Minegishi S, Tamura K, Okano Y, et al. Utility and feasibility of a new programmable home blood pressure monitoring device for the assessment of nighttime blood pressure. Clin Exp Nephrol. 2009;13:480–5.
8. Ishikawa J, Hoshide S, Eguchi K, Ishikawa S, Shimada K, Kario K, et al. Nighttime home blood pressure and the risk of hypertensive target organ damage. Hypertension. 2012;60:921–8.
9. Stergiou GS, Nasothimiou EG, Destounis A, Poulidakis E, Evagelou I, Tzamouranis D. Assessment of the diurnal blood pressure profile and detection of non-dippers based on home or ambulatory monitoring. Am J Hypertens. 2012;25(9):974–8.
10. Stergiou GS, Triantafyllidou E, Cholidou K, Kollias A, Destounis A, Nasothimiou EG, et al. Asleep home blood pressure monitoring in obstructive sleep apnea: a pilot study. Blood Press Monit. 2013;18(1):21–6.
11. Andreadis EA, Agaliotis G, Kollias A, Kolyvas G, Achimastos A, Stergiou GS. Night-time home versus ambulatory blood pressure in determining target organ damage. J Hypertens. 2016;34(3):438–44.
12. Lindroos AS, Johansson JK, Puukka PJ, Kantola I, Salomaa V, Juhanoja EP, et al. The association between home vs. ambulatory night-time blood pressure and end-organ damage in the general population. J Hypertens. 2016;34(9):1730–7.
13. Lindroos AS, Jula AM, Puukka PJ, Kantola I, Salomaa V, Juhanoja E, et al. Comparison of acceptability of traditional and novel blood pressure measurement methods. Am J Hypertens. 2016;29:679–83.
14. Kario K, Hoshide S, Shimizu M, Yano Y, Eguchi K, Ishikawa J, et al. Effect of dosing time of angiotensin II receptor blockade titrated by self-measured blood pressure recordings on cardiorenal protection in hypertensives: the Japan morning surge-target organ protection (J-TOP) study. J Hypertens. 2010;28:1574–83.
15. Kario K, Tomitani N, Kanegae H, Ishii H, Uchiyama K, Yamagiwa K, et al. Comparative effects of an angiotensin II receptor blocker (ARB)/diuretic vs. ARB/calcium-channel blocker combination on uncontrolled nocturnal hypertension evaluated by information and communication technology-based nocturnal home blood pressure monitoring - the NOCTURNE study. Circ J. 2017;81:948–57.
16. Fujiwara T, Tomitani N, Kanegae H, Kario K. Comparative effects of valsartan plus either cilnidipine or hydrochlorothiazide on home morning blood pressure surge evaluated by information and communication technology-based nocturnal home blood pressure monitoring. J Clin Hypertens. 2018;20:159–67.
17. McGowan NJ, Gough K, Padfield PL. Nocturnal dipping is reproducible in the long term. Blood Press Monit. 2009;14:185–9.
18. Omboni S, Parati G, Palatini P, Vanasia A, Muiesan ML, Cuspidi C, et al. Reproducibility and clinical value of nocturnal hypotension: prospective evidence from the SAMPLE study. Study on ambulatory monitoring of pressure and lisinopril evaluation. J Hypertens. 1998;16:733–8.

19. Kollias A, Ntineri A, Stergiou GS. Association of night-time home blood pressure with night-time ambulatory blood pressure and target-organ damage: a systematic review and meta-analysis. J Hypertens. 2017;35(3):442–52.
20. Routledge FS, McFetridge-Durdle JA, Dean CR. Canadian hypertension society. Night-time blood pressure patterns and target organ damage: a review. Can J Cardiol. 2007;23(2):132–8.
21. Kario K, Hamasaki H. Nocturnal blood pressure surge behind morning surge in obstructive sleep apnea syndrome: another phenotype of systemic hemodynamic Atherothrombotic syndrome. J Clin Hypertens (Greenwich). 2015;17(9):682–5.
22. Kario K. Essential manual on perfect 24-hour blood pressure management from morning to nocturnal hypertension: up-to-date for anticipation medicine. Tokyo, Japan: Wiley; 2015. p. 1–309.
23. Ishikawa J, Shimizu M, Sugiyama Edison E, Yano Y, Hoshide S, Eguchi K, et al. Assessment of the reductions in night-time blood pressure and dipping induced by antihypertensive medication using a home blood pressure monitor. J Hypertens. 2014;32(1):82–9.
24. Kollias A, Andreadis E, Agaliotis G, Kolyvas GN, Achimastos A, Stergiou GS. The optimal night-time home blood pressure monitoring schedule: agreement with ambulatory blood pressure and association with organ damage. J Hypertens. 2018;36(2):243–9.
25. Kario K, Kuwabara M, Hoshide S, Nagai M, Shimpo M. Effects of nighttime single-dose administration of vasodilating vs sympatholytic antihypertensive agents on sleep blood pressure in hypertensive patients with sleep apnea syndrome. J Clin Hypertens (Greenwich). 2014;16(6):459–66.
26. Kario K, Hoshide S, Haimoto H, et al. Sleep blood pressure self- measured at home as a novel determinant of organ damage: Japan morning surge home blood pressure (J-HOP) study. J Clin Hypertens. 2015;17:340–8.
27. Tabara Y, Matsumoto T, Murase K, Nagashima S, Hirai T, Kosugi S, et al. Seasonal variation in nocturnal home blood pressure fall: the Nagahama study. Hypertens Res. 2018;41(3):198–208.
28. Stergiou GS, Myrsilidi A, Kollias A, Destounis A, Roussias L, Kalogeropoulos P. Seasonal variation in meteorological parameters and office, ambulatory and home blood pressure: predicting factors and clinical implications. Hypertens Res. 2015;38:869–75.
29. Kario K. Nocturnal hypertension: new technology and evidence. Hypertension. 2018;71:997–1009.
30. Beltman FW, Heesen WF, Smit AJ, May JF, Lie KI, Meyboom-de Jong B. Acceptance and side effects of ambulatory blood pressure monitoring: evaluation of a new technology. J Hum Hypertens. 1996;10(Suppl 3):S39–42.
31. Mallion JM, de Gaudemaris R, Baguet JP, Azzouzi L, Quesada JL, Sauzeau C, et al. Acceptability and tolerance of ambulatory blood pressure measurement in the hypertensive patient. Blood Press Monit. 1996;1(3):197–203.
32. Alessi A, Alessi CR, Piana ER, Assis M, Oliveira LR, Cunha CL. Influence of quality of sleep on the nocturnal decline in blood pressure during ambulatory blood pressure monitoring. Arq Bras Cardiol. 2002;78(2):212–23.
33. Imai Y, Asayama K, Fujiwara S, Saito K, Sato H, Haga T, et al. Development and evaluation of a home nocturnal blood pressure monitoring system using a wrist-cuff device. Blood Press Monit. 2018;23(6):318–26.

Home Blood Pressure Monitoring in Children, Pregnancy, and Chronic Kidney Disease

13

Anastasios Kollias, Andrew Shennan, Rajiv Agarwal, Angeliki Ntineri, and George S. Stergiou

13.1 Home Blood Pressure Monitoring in Children

A. Kollias A. Ntineri, and G. S. Stergiou

Conventional office blood pressure (BP) measurement has been the cornerstone for screening and evaluation of hypertension in children. The recent European Society of Hypertension (ESH) and US guidelines for pediatric hypertension have put considerable emphasis on the methodology of office BP measurements stressing the role of standardized measurement conditions, use of appropriate validated monitors and cuff sizes, and performing multiple measurements [1, 2]. Despite the detailed instructions by the guidelines, it is well recognized that assessment solely based on office BP measurements frequently leads to inaccurate diagnosis, mainly due to the white-coat and masked hypertension phenomena which are common in children as

A. Kollias · A. Ntineri · G. S. Stergiou (✉)
Hypertension Center STRIDE-7, National and Kapodistrian University of Athens, School of Medicine, Third Department of Medicine, Sotiria Hospital, Athens, Greece
e-mail: gstergi@med.uoa.gr

A. Shennan
Department of Women and Children's Health, School of Life Course Sciences, FoLSM, King's College, London, UK
e-mail: andrew.shennan@kcl.ac.uk

R. Agarwal
Indiana University School of Medicine and Richard L. Roudebush VA Medical Center, Indianapolis, USA
e-mail: ragarwal@iu.edu

© The Editor(s), under exclusive license to Springer Nature Switzerland AG 2020
G. S. Stergiou et al. (eds.), *Home Blood Pressure Monitoring*,
Updates in Hypertension and Cardiovascular Protection,
https://doi.org/10.1007/978-3-030-23065-4_13

in the adults [1–3]. Thus, it is currently recommended that documentation of elevated BP out of the office is needed to confirm the diagnosis of hypertension, mainly using ambulatory BP monitoring [1, 2].

Ambulatory BP monitoring has a central role in the accurate diagnosis of hypertension in children due to the existing and accumulating evidence on its clinical and research value [1, 2]. On the other hand the potential of home BP monitoring in the evaluation of pediatric hypertension remains largely unrecognized and inadequately investigated [4, 5]. However, the available evidence suggests that home BP monitoring appears to have several advantages over both office and ambulatory BP monitoring, including convenience and the ability to obtain multiple measurements in the usual environment of the individual over several days, weeks or months [1–5]. It is important to mention that home BP monitoring is already being used in children as a part of routine clinical practice, as shown by surveys in the USA, Canada, and Germany, which report that more than 70% of pediatric nephrologists utilize home BP monitoring in children with hypertension or renal disease, and 64% of them consider home measurements more important than office measurements [6, 7].

Despite the fact that in children the research evidence on ambulatory BP is stronger than for home BP monitoring, the preliminary evidence for home BP monitoring in this population is in line with that in adults showing that: (a) the reproducibility of home BP monitoring is superior to that of office BP measurements and close to that of ambulatory BP monitoring [8, 9], (b) there is close agreement between home and ambulatory BP monitoring in diagnosing hypertension phenotypes within the range of 80–85% [10, 11], (c) the association of home BP monitoring with several indices of preclinical target-organ damage, mainly left ventricular mass index, appears to be similar to ambulatory BP monitoring and superior to office BP measurements [11, 12].

Automated oscillometric BP measuring devices are almost exclusively used for ambulatory and home BP monitoring. However, the published evidence on the accuracy of automated oscillometric BP monitors in children is limited. A recent systematic review identified 31 formal validation studies of oscillometric BP monitors in children, of which 42% were published a decade ago or longer [13]. Of these 31 studies, 16 evaluated devices for office BP measurements, five of which failed; nine evaluated ambulatory BP monitoring devices, of which three failed; and six evaluated home BP monitoring devices, one of which failed [13].

Normalcy data for home BP in children and adolescents have been derived from a single cross-sectional school-based study [14] in 778 children and adolescents in Greece and have been adopted by the ESH and US pediatric guidelines as percentile tables according to gender and height (Table 13.1). In this study, home BP monitoring was performed using an electronic (oscillometric) device (Omron 705 IT) which has been validated for accuracy specifically in children and adolescents [15]. It should be mentioned that in children and adolescents, the relationship between office, home, and ambulatory BP thresholds provided by the widely used normalcy tables differs from that in the adults. In contrast to data in adults in whom home BP values are similar to those of daytime ambulatory BP, in children and adolescents systolic home BP (and less so diastolic BP) is significantly lower than daytime ambulatory BP [16]. This disparity is probably attributed to the higher level of physical activity during the day in the younger population. Moreover, there is a trend for office BP to be lower than

Table 13.1 Normalcy tables for home blood pressure (mmHg) in children and adolescents by gender and height (with permission from [14])

Height (cm)	N	Percentiles for boys ($n = 347$)		N	Percentiles for girls ($n = 420$)	
		50th	95th		50th	95th
120–129	23	105/64	119/76	36	101/64	119/74
130–139	51	108/64	121/77	51	103/64	120/76
140–149	39	110/65	125/77	61	105/65	122/77
150–159	41	112/65	126/78	71	108/66	123/77
160–169	45	115/65	128/78	148	110/66	124/78
170–179	91	117/66	132/78	46	112/66	125/79
180–189	57	121/67	134/79	7	114/67	128/80

Table 13.2 Instructions for home blood pressure monitoring in children and adolescents (permission from [5])

Devices
- Use automated electronic (oscillometric) upper-arm devices that have been successfully validated specifically in children
- Ensure the appropriate cuff size for the individual's arm circumference is utilized
- Select devices equipped with automated memory or PC link capacity when available

Conditions
- Measurements may be taken by parents of young children, or self-measurements may be appropriate for some adolescents
- Perform measurements in a quiet room after 5 min of rest in the seated position with back supported and arm resting at heart level

Schedule
- Monitor home blood pressure for no less than 3 routine school days but preferably 6–7 days
- Obtain duplicate morning and evening measurements (with 1 min intervals) on each day BP is monitored

Interpretation
- Calculate the average of all measurements after discarding the first day
- Evaluate the average value using the available normalcy data for home blood pressure in children
- Average home blood pressure ≥95th percentile for gender and height indicates home hypertension

home or daytime ambulatory BP in the younger age subgroups, but this difference is progressively eliminated with increasing age, apart from systolic BP in boys [16].

Instructions for home BP monitoring in children and adolescents are shown in Table 13.2 [5]. Use of automated electronic (oscillometric) upper-arm devices that have been successfully validated specifically in children is recommended. Moreover, using devices with automated memory or PC-link capacity avoids potential reporting bias with over- or underreporting of home BP readings. A 6- to 7-day (minimum 3-day) schedule with duplicate morning (before drug intake if treated) and evening home BP measurements taken in the sitting position after few minutes rest is currently suggested since this is in line with the recommendation in adults and this has been validated in children and adolescents [17]. The average value of all measurements after discarding the first day is used for the BP assessment. This schedule should be performed for the initial diagnosis in children with suspected hypertension as complementary to ambulatory BP monitoring, and also before each follow-up visit to the doctor in children with treated hypertension. In the long-term monitoring of children treated for hypertension, 1–2 home measurements per week between office visits, or even less frequent, might suffice [5].

In conclusion, home BP monitoring in children appears to be superior to office BP due to several advantages, including the detection of white-coat and masked hypertension, lack of observer error and bias, and higher reproducibility. However, since the current evidence for ambulatory BP monitoring in children is much stronger, this method should have the primary role in diagnosis, with home BP monitoring being used if ambulatory monitoring is not available or not tolerated. Data on the optimal home BP monitoring schedule, and normalcy tables with thresholds (percentiles) for home hypertension diagnosis are now available but the evidence on the relationship with preclinical target-organ damage and validation of electronic home monitors in children is limited. Accumulating data will probably allow home BP monitoring to acquire an evidence-based role in wide clinical application in children and adolescents in near future.

13.2   Home Blood Pressure Monitoring in Pregnancy

A. Shennan

Measuring BP in pregnancy has unique importance and its own specific challenges [18]. It is fundamental to both detecting and managing hypertension in pregnancy, which can have acute implications for both mother and baby. Hypertension maybe a sign of preeclampsia, a leading cause of maternal mortality (14%) and preterm birth (20%) globally [19]. Preeclampsia, characterized by hypertension, is often asymptomatic, even if severe, and BP measurement is the hallmark of identification. One-quarter of all stillbirths and neonatal deaths are attributed to this disease in low and middle income countries. If left unrecognized, life-threatening disease invariably ensues, usually within 2 weeks. Measuring BP will identify those who need monitoring and delivery, and indicate those who require therapy to reduce the risk of cerebrovascular events. When correctly managed, preeclampsia deaths are largely avoidable [20]. The implications of over or missed diagnosis are substantial and therefore correct BP measurement is key to safe management.

BP should be measured at every antenatal visit. However, even antenatal schedules may not be sufficiently frequent to identify fulminant preeclampsia where onset and progress can be rapid and often asymptomatic. The potential for home monitoring to assist in identification and management is therefore substantial.

Care in technique and correct cuff size is similar to all patients, but specifically aortocaval compression should be avoided when lying supine in the third trimester by left lateral tilt. Sitting is an appropriate instruction for those using home monitors. Korotkoff fifth sound should be used for auscultation in determining diastolic BP [21] if used in clinic to compare with home assessment to elucidate white-coat effects. The vasodilatation of pregnancy does not alter the accuracy of the fifth Korotkoff sound, and home BP devices should be validated to this diastolic endpoint. Digit preference is common among midwives at initial assessment and threshold avoidance must be avoided given the possible severe implications of even mild hypertension in pregnancy. Home monitoring helps eliminate these errors.

Oscillometric monitors do under record the BP in preeclampsia, and often by significant amounts (>10 mmHg). This is related to the decreased arterial compliance, the reduced intra-vascular volume in preeclampsia and the interstitial edema which affect the amplitude and detection of the oscillometric waveform [18]. As each algorithm is unique, every device should be validated in pregnancy, once the device has passed an adult validation. Some companies have a generic algorithm that is suited to pregnancy (e.g., Microlife and Omron) and therefore have a few models suited for use, and most of these are appropriate for home monitoring. Accuracy assessment in pregnancy must include both women with preeclampsia ($n = 15$) and women with a range of BPs ($n = 30$). The Cradle VSA also has a traffic light warning system for both high and low BP, where the shock index (Heart rate/Systolic BP) has been shown to reliable detect shock associated with obstetric hemorrhage and sepsis [22]. The traffic light can be useful for home monitoring as provides a simple action point for patients. The Cradle VSA can also be used as a manometer with an auscultatory technique if clinicians want to confirm unusual results. The devices that have been validated for use in pregnancy are shown in Table 13.3.

BP thresholds are similar to non-pregnant values. Levels over 140 mmHg systolic and 90 mmHg diastolic are significant. Measurements at home in pregnancy appear similar to that in clinic, so management thresholds can be similar, but white-coat hypertension is still common [23]. The physiological BP fall in pregnancy does mean these thresholds are more significant (higher standard deviation above normal) in early pregnancy. However the importance of BP is greater in later pregnancy, and a single threshold remains diagnostic for pragmatic reasons. In acute control, systolic BP should be kept under 150 mmHg to avoid stroke. Postpartum thresholds should be the same. The need and benefit of treating mild to moderate hypertension in pregnancy is controversial, as the reduction in placental perfusion may be detrimental. For every 10 mmHg drop in BP, there is nearly a 150 g reduction in birthweight [24]. BP control does not alter the course of preeclampsia and can mask disease progression. It is therefore not necessary to acutely treat BP under 150/100 mmHg.

Hypertension in pregnancy is a risk factor for later cardiovascular disease. There is a doubling of risk of stroke, ischemic heart disease and venous thromboembolic disease up to 14 years later, and a fourfold increase risk of hypertension in later life [25]. Cardiovascular risk assessment should occur postpartum, including BP assessment, to instigate lifestyle modification and other prophylactic therapy as necessary

Table 13.3 Devices validated in pregnancy

Manufacturer	Device model
Omron	MIT[a], MIT Elite[a], Hem 705CP[a], M7[a]
Microlife	Watch BP Home[a], BP 3BTO-A[a], BP 3AS1-2[a], Cradle VSA[a]
Welch Allyn	Spot Vital Sign
Dinamap	ProCare 400

[a]Implies suitable for home use

[26]. The advantage of home monitoring is that the same device can be used to ascertain postpartum risk.

Low dose aspirin (75–150 mg) should be prescribed to women at risk of pre-eclampsia. This includes women with underlying hypertension. New algorithms to determine risk rely on automated but validated BP equipment to accurately ascertain who will benefit from aspirin [27]. In women with uncertain booking BP, or possible white-coat hypertension, home monitoring may aid in targeting aspirin prophylaxis.

Both home and ambulatory BP monitoring have been shown to more accurately characterize BP in pregnancy as in non-pregnant individuals. Monitoring at home is acceptable to women, and results in fewer antenatal visits overall while improving surveillance [28]. This has resulted in improved prediction in early pregnancy and potentially better management when deciding on therapeutic decisions in pregnancy where the fetal exposure of drugs must also be considered. The widespread use of ambulatory monitoring has not occurred, but increasing use of home monitoring increases surveillance. Home monitors must be validated for use in pregnancy to avoid false reassurance of inaccurate devices.

13.3 Home Blood Pressure Monitoring in Chronic Kidney Disease

R. Agarwal

For making a diagnosis of hypertension, ambulatory BP monitoring is considered the reference standard. Among patients with chronic kidney disease (CKD), using ambulatory BP monitoring as the reference standard, compared to clinic BP measurements made with strict adherence to technique or even when they are measured using a standardized methodology, home BP monitoring has a better ability to diagnose lack or control of hypertension [29]. A formal evaluation of the diagnostic test performance demonstrated a higher area under the receiver operating characteristic curve of home BP compared to clinic BP [29]. One week averaged home BP of >140/80 mmHg associates with awake ambulatory BP of >130/80 mmHg. The latter is considered hypertensive by the newer guidelines. The threshold of 140 mmHg systolic or 80 mmHg diastolic BP have a sensitivity of >80% and specificity of >80% to diagnose hypertension; accordingly, these thresholds may be useful for clinical decision-making.

Studies suggest that home BP measurements are of prognostic significance. As examples, among 77 patients with type 1 diabetic kidney disease, at mean follow-up of about 6 years compared to office BP, home BP was a stronger predictor of decline in GFR [30]. Agarwal and Andersen compared the prognostic value of clinic and home BP monitoring (3 measurements/day for 1 week) in a cohort of 217 mostly male veterans with CKD [31]. In this study home BP was prognostically superior to clinic BP and predicted end-stage renal disease (ESRD) independently of other risk factors. Masked hypertension, in this study, associated with an increased risk of ESRD [31]. In comparison to white-coat hypertension, the risk of ESRD with sustained hypertension was much higher. These data attest to the value of home BP monitoring in patients with CKD.

Peridialysis BPs that are routinely obtained in the dialysis unit before and after dialysis without using a specified technique may be useful in a qualitative sense but cannot be used to determine interdialytic BP [32]. For example, among 70 patients on chronic hemodialysis, who underwent ambulatory BP monitoring for the diagnosis of hypertension, Agarwal and Lewis found that the agreement limits between pre/postdialysis BP and ambulatory BP are sufficiently wide to preclude determination of ambulatory BP [33]. Predialysis BP of >150/85 mmHg has a >80% sensitivity but is not sufficiently specific in diagnosing hypertension. Postdialysis BP of >130/75 mmHg also has >80% sensitivity but is not sufficiently specific in diagnosing hypertension when the reference standard of ambulatory BP monitoring is used. Similar results were obtained in a meta-analysis, which found poor agreement between ambulatory BP recordings and pre/postdialysis BP measurements [34]. Cohort studies demonstrate that home BP recordings are superior to peridialysis BP measurements in predicting all-cause mortality [35, 36].

To best estimate the usual level of BP in a patient with ESRD on long-term hemodialysis, the timing and the number of BP measured at home is of critical importance. When should BP be measured and how many measurements should be made requires an understanding of the BP patterns among these patients [37]. Typically, among patients with ESRD, hemodialysis is carried out 3 times a week. This means that there are 2–3 days between treatments when dialysis is not administered. Home systolic BP increases linearly by about 4 mmHg every 10 h for the first 2 days (Fig. 13.1) [37]. Thereafter, BP plateaus (Fig. 13.1) [37]. During the dialysis treatment volume removal—ultrafiltration—results in a large decline in systolic BP. This decline in systolic BP is proportional to the volume removed. Therefore, those patients who have a large interdialytic weight gain will also have a large decline in systolic BP during the dialysis treatment. It is evident that these patients will also have the largest increments in interdialytic BP. Conversely, those patients who have little change in an interdialytic weight gain will also have the smallest intradialytic and interdialytic excursions in the linear component of their BP (Fig. 13.2). At approximately 24 h from the end of dialysis treatment, systolic BP in the high weight gainers and low weight gainers is similar [37]. However, for diastolic BP this occurs at approximately 36 h. Therefore, it is recommended that home BP be measured twice daily, at bedtime and on waking up, after the midweek dialysis for 4 days. This will allow sampling of a wide range of BP which when compared with the interdialytic 44-h ambulatory BP monitoring has the best agreement. In one study that validated home BP recordings against 44-h ambulatory BP measurements it was noted that home systolic BP of 150/80 mmHg had both 80% sensitivity and 80% specificity in diagnosing interdialytic ambulatory hypertension among long-term hemodialysis patients [37].

In a study from Brazil, patients were randomized either to management of hypertension using a strategy using predialysis BP or BP measured by the patients at home [38]. The primary endpoint of the study was to examine the change from baseline in 44 h interdialytic ambulatory BP. It was noted that only in the group that

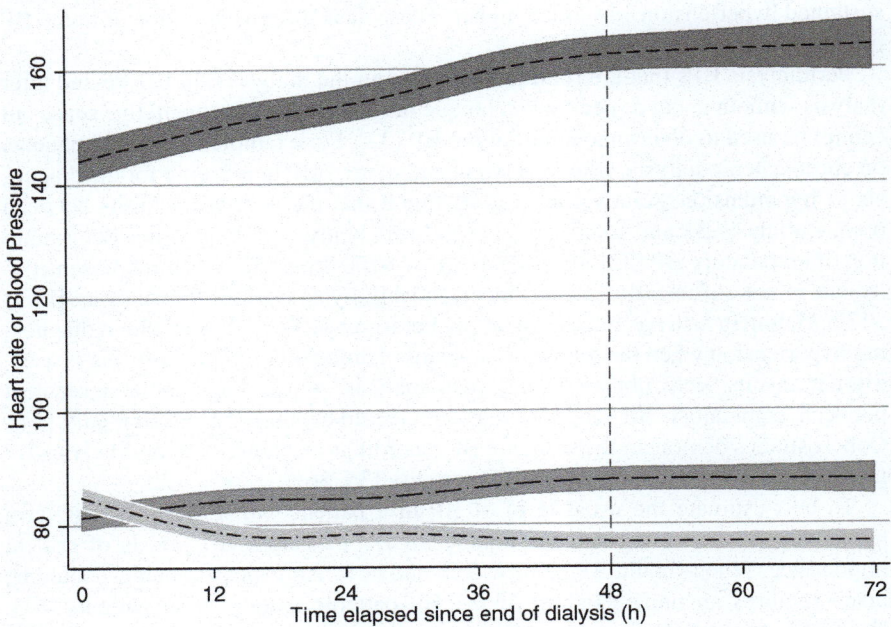

Fig. 13.1 Non-linear relationships of home blood pressure and heart rate over an interdialytic interval modeled using restricted cubic splines. After about 48 h (vertical line) the changes in home BP and heart rate plateau. Pulse pressure is amplified over time between dialysis treatments (with permission from [37])

was randomized to home BP measurements there was a significant decline in ambulatory BP; predialysis BP measurement-managed group had no such change [38]. This study was the first to demonstrate that home BP monitoring is important in managing hypertension in the hemodialysis patients.

Home BP monitoring can also be useful to decide when a hemodialysis patient does not need antihypertensive drugs. To ascertain the appropriateness of antihypertensive therapy, Bishu et al. conducted a prospective study in which they discontinued antihypertensive drugs in hemodialysis patients and performed 44-h interdialytic ambulatory BP monitoring and measured left ventricular mass and inferior vena cava by echocardiography [39]. Home BP was monitored weekly during washout. An average of 2.3 medications were tapered and discontinued in 41 black participants (age 56 years, 46% men, 54% diabetes mellitus, duration of dialysis 5.3 years). Thirty-three of 41 (80%) of the patients became hypertensive but 8 (20%) remained normotensive at 3–5 weeks. Those patients who remained normotensive had lower home BP at baseline (135/76 vs. 147/85 mmHg) and had a lower left ventricular mass index (115 vs. 146 g/m^2). None of the normotensives were volume overloaded in contrast to 12% of the hypertensives. Thus, patients with well controlled home BP who have no left ventricular hypertrophy may have a cautious withdrawal of their antihypertensive drugs.

In the hemodialysis patients randomized to atenolol or lisinopril (HDPAL) trial, patients were managed using home BP measurements every month for a 12-month

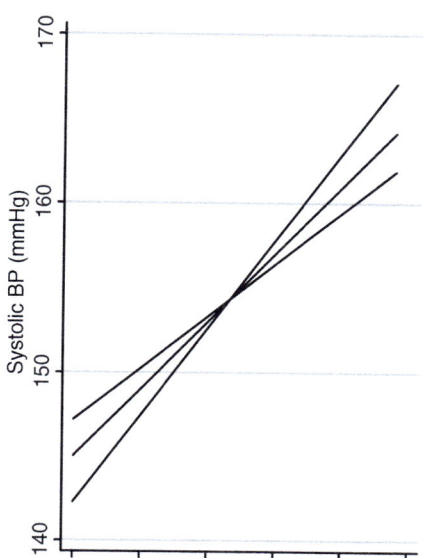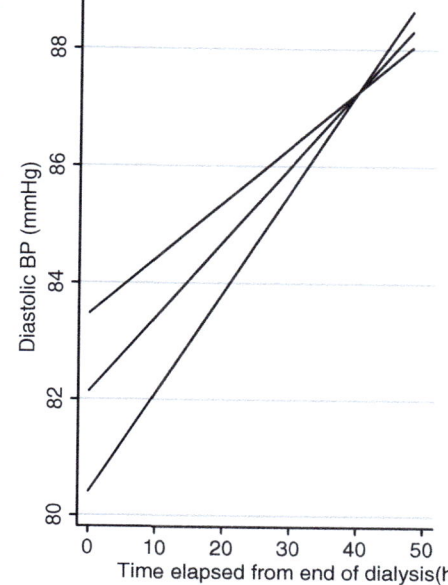

Fig. 13.2 Effect of interdialytic weight gain on home BP changes. Home BP rises 0.4 mmHg/h systolic and 0.13 mmHg/h diastolic in the interdialytic period in those who gain median weight (2.35 kg over 2 days). In those who gain more weight the intercept systolic BP is lower (by 1.6 mmHg/kg systolic and 1.0 mmHg/kg diastolic) but the rate of rise is steeper (by 0.07 mmHg/h/kg systolic and 0.025 mmHg/h/kg diastolic). In those who gain less weight have a slower rate of rise in interdialytic BP. The point where BP is least influenced by weight gain is about 24 h for systolic and 40 h of diastolic BP. Thus, sampling home BP over each third of time elapsed after dialysis will give the most reliable estimates of interdialytic ambulatory BP (with permission from [37])

period [40]. In this study the target home BP was 140/90 mmHg and 100 patients were randomized to each group. The reductions from baseline in 44-h interdialytic ambulatory BP within 3 months in this randomized interventional trial were approximately 15–20 mm systolic for either group, attesting to the value of home BP monitoring in the management of these patients.

We therefore recommend measuring BP twice daily—at bedtime and on waking up—after a mid-week dialysis treatment for four consecutive days [41]. We attempt to target mean home BP measured in this way to <140/90 mmHg. By extrapolation, among patients on peritoneal dialysis, we recommend measuring BP twice daily—at bedtime and on waking up—for four consecutive days.

References

1. Lurbe E, Agabiti-Rosei E, Cruickshank JK, Dominiczak A, Erdine S, Hirth A, et al. 2016 European Society of Hypertension guidelines for the management of high blood pressure in children and adolescents. J Hypertens. 2016;34:1887–920.

2. Flynn JT, Kaelber DC, Baker-Smith CM, Blowey D, Carroll AE, Daniels SR, et al. Clinical practice guideline for screening and management of high blood pressure in children and adolescents. Pediatrics. 2017;140:pii: e20171904.
3. Stergiou GS, Alamara CV, Vazeou A, Stefanidis CJ. Office and out-of-office blood pressure measurement in children and adolescents. Blood Press Monit. 2004;9:293–6.
4. Stergiou GS, Ntineri A, Kollias A, Stambolliu E, Kapogiannis A, Vazeou A, et al. Home blood pressure monitoring in pediatric hypertension: the US perspective and a plan for action. Hypertens Res. 2018;41:662–8.
5. Stergiou GS, Ntineri A. Methodology and applicability of home blood pressure monitoring in children and adolescents. In: Flynn J, Ingelfinger J, Redwine K, editors. Pediatric Hypertension. Cham: Springer; 2018. p. 305–21. https://doi.org/10.1007/978-3-319-31107-4_45.
6. Bald M, Hoyer PF. Measurement of blood pressure at home: survey among pediatric nephrologists. Pediatr Nephrol. 2001;16:1058–62.
7. Woroniecki RP, Flynn JT. How are hypertensive children evaluated and managed? A survey of North American pediatric nephrologists. Pediatr Nephrol. 2005;20:791–7.
8. Stergiou GS, Alamara CV, Salgami EV, Vaindirlis IN, Dacou-Voutetakis C, Mountokalakis TD. Reproducibility of home and ambulatory blood pressure in children and adolescents. Blood Press Monit. 2005;10:143–7.
9. Stergiou GS, Nasothimiou EG, Giovas PP, Rarra VC. Long-term reproducibility of home vs. office blood pressure in children and adolescents: the Arsakeion school study. Hypertens Res. 2009;32:311–5.
10. Stergiou GS, Nasothimiou E, Giovas P, Kapoyiannis A, Vazeou A. Diagnosis of hypertension in children and adolescents based on home versus ambulatory blood pressure monitoring. J Hypertens. 2008;26:1556–62.
11. Stergiou GS, Giovas PP, Kollias A, Rarra VC, Papagiannis J, Georgakopoulos D, et al. Relationship of home blood pressure with target-organ damage in children and adolescents. Hypertens Res. 2011;34:640–4.
12. Kollias A, Dafni M, Poulidakis E, Ntineri A, Stergiou GS. Out-of-office blood pressure and target organ damage in children and adolescents: a systematic review and meta-analysis. J Hypertens. 2014;32:2315–31.
13. Stergiou GS, Boubouchairopoulou N, Kollias A. Accuracy of automated blood pressure measurement in children: evidence, issues, and perspectives. Hypertension. 2017;69:1000–6.
14. Stergiou GS, Yiannes NG, Rarra VC, Panagiotakos DB. Home blood pressure normalcy in children and adolescents: the Arsakeion School study. J Hypertens. 2007;25:1375–9.
15. Stergiou GS, Yiannes NG, Rarra VC. Validation of the Omron 705 IT oscillometric device for home blood pressure measurement in children and adolescents: the Arsakion School study. Blood Press Monit. 2006;11:229–34.
16. Stergiou GS, Karpettas N, Panagiotakos DB, Vazeou A. Comparison of office, ambulatory and home blood pressure in children and adolescents on the basis of normalcy tables. J Hum Hypertens. 2011;25:218–23.
17. Stergiou GS, Christodoulakis G, Giovas P, Lourida P, Alamara C, Roussias LG. Home blood pressure monitoring in children: how many measurements are needed? Am J Hypertens. 2008;21:633–8.
18. Nathan HL, Duhig K, Hezelgrave NL, Chappell LC, Shennan AH. Blood pressure measurement in pregnancy. Obstet Gynaecol. 2015;17:91–8.
19. Duley L. The global impact of pre-eclampsia and eclampsia. Semin Perinatol. 2009;33:130–7.
20. Shennan AH, Green M, Chappell LC. Maternal deaths in the UK: pre-eclampsia deaths are avoidable. Lancet. 2017;389:582–4.
21. Shennan A, Gupta M, Halligan A, Taylor DJ, de Swiet M. Lack of reproducibility in pregnancy of Korotkoff phase IV as measured by mercury sphygmomanometry. Lancet. 1996;347:139–42.
22. Nathan HL, Vousden N, Lawley E, de Greeff A, Hezelgrave NL, Sloan N, et al. Development and evaluation of a novel vital signs alert device for use in pregnancy in low-resource settings. BMJ Innov. 2018;4:192–8.

23. Tucker KL, Bankhead C, Hodgkinson J, Roberts N, Stevens R, Heneghan C, et al. How do home and clinic blood pressure readings compare in pregnancy? Hypertension. 2018;72:686–94.
24. von Dadelszen P, Ornstein MP, Bull SB, Logan AG, Koren G, Magee LA. Fall in mean arterial pressure and fetal growth restriction in pregnancy hypertension: a meta-analysis. Lancet. 2000;355:87–92.
25. Bellamy L, Casas JP, Hingorami AD, Williams DJ. Preeclampsia and risk of cardiovascular disease and cancer in later life: systematic review and meta-analysis. BMJ. 2007;335:974.
26. Magee L, von Dadelszen P. Preeclampsia and increased cardiovascular risk. BMJ. 2007;335:945–6.
27. Rolnik DL, Wright D, Poon LC, O'Gorman N, Syngelaki A, de Paco Matallana C, et al. Aspirin versus placebo in pregnancies at high risk for preterm preeclampsia. N Engl J Med. 2017;377:613–22.
28. Ross-McGill H, Hewison J, Hirst J, Dowswell T, Holt A, Brunskill P, et al. Antenatal home blood pressure monitoring: a pilot randomised controlled trial. BJOG. 2000;107:217–21.
29. Andersen MJ, Khawandi W, Agarwal R. Home blood pressure monitoring in CKD. Am J Kidney Dis. 2005;45:994–1001.
30. Rave K, Bender R, Heise T, Sawicki PT. Value of blood pressure self-monitoring as a predictor of progression of diabetic nephropathy. J Hypertens. 1999;17:597–601.
31. Agarwal R, Andersen MJ. Prognostic importance of clinic and home blood pressure recordings in patients with chronic kidney disease. Kidney Int. 2006;69:406–11.
32. Santos SF, Mendes RB, Santos CA, Dorigo D, Peixoto AJ. Profile of interdialytic blood pressure in hemodialysis patients. Am J Nephrol. 2003;23:96–105.
33. Agarwal R, Lewis RR. Prediction of hypertension in chronic hemodialysis patients. Kidney Int. 2001;60:1982–9.
34. Agarwal R, Peixoto AJ, Santos SF, Zoccali C. Pre and post dialysis blood pressures are imprecise estimates of interdialytic ambulatory blood pressure. Clin J Am Soc Nephrol. 2006;1:389–98.
35. Alborzi P, Patel N, Agarwal R. Home blood pressures are of greater prognostic value than hemodialysis unit recordings. Clin J Am Soc Nephrol. 2007;2:1228–34.
36. Agarwal R. Blood pressure and mortality among hemodialysis patients. Hypertension. 2010;55:762–8.
37. Agarwal R, Light RP. Chronobiology of arterial hypertension in hemodialysis patients: implications for home blood pressure monitoring. Am J Kidney Dis. 2009;54:693–701.
38. da Silva GV, de Barros S, Abensur H, Ortega KC, Mion D Jr. Cochrane renal group prospective trial register: CRG060800146. Home blood pressure monitoring in blood pressure control among haemodialysis patients: An open randomized clinical trial. Nephrol Dial Transplant. 2009;24:3805–11.
39. Bishu K, Gricz KM, Chewaka S, Agarwal R. Appropriateness of antihypertensive drug therapy in hemodialysis patients. Clin J Am Soc Nephrol. 2006;1:820–4.
40. Agarwal R, Sinha AD, Pappas MK, Abraham TN, Tegegne GG. Hypertension in hemodialysis patients treated with atenolol or lisinopril: a randomized controlled trial. Nephrol Dial Transplant. 2014;29:672–81.
41. Agarwal R, Andersen MJ, Light RP. Location not quantity of blood pressure measurements predicts mortality in hemodialysis patients. Am J Nephrol. 2007;28:210–7.

Home Blood Pressure Variability

14

Gianfranco Parati, Juan Eugenio Ochoa, Yutaka Imai,
Anastasios Kollias, Efstathios Manios, Takayoshi Ohkubo,
Kazuomi Kario, George S. Stergiou, and Grzegorz Bilo

G. Parati (✉)
Department of Medicine and Surgery, University of Milano-Bicocca, Milan, Italy

Istituto Auxologico Italiano, IRCCS, Department of Cardiovascular, Neural and Metabolic
Sciences, Milan, Italy
e-mail: gianfranco.parati@unimib.it

J. E. Ochoa
Istituto Auxologico Italiano, IRCCS, Department of Cardiovascular Neural and Metabolic
Sciences, Milan, Italy

Y. Imai
Tohoku Institute for Management of Blood Pressure, Sendai, Japan
e-mail: yutaka.imai.d6@tohoku.ac.jp

A. Kollias · G. S. Stergiou
Hypertension Center STRIDE-7, National and Kapodistrian University of Athens, School of
Medicine, Third Department of Medicine, Sotiria Hospital, Athens, Greece
e-mail: gstergi@med.uoa.gr

E. Manios
Department of Clinical Therapeutics, National and Kapodistrian University of Athens,
Medical School, Alexandra Hospital, Athens, Greece

T. Ohkubo
Department of Hygiene and Public Health, Teikyo University School of Medicine,
Tokyo, Japan

Tohoku Institute for Management of Blood Pressure, Sendai, Japan
e-mail: tohkubo@med.teikyo-u.ac.jp

K. Kario
Division of Cardiovascular Medicine, Department of Medicine, Jichi Medical University
School of Medicine (JMU), Tochigi, Japan
e-mail: kkario@jichi.ac.jp

G. Bilo
Istituto Auxologico Italiano, IRCCS, Department of Cardiovascular Neural and Metabolic
Sciences, Milan, Italy

Department of Medicine and Surgery, University of Milano-Bicocca, Milan, Italy
e-mail: g.bilo@auxologico.it

143

14.1   Introduction

Blood pressure (BP) values change significantly over time as a result of the interaction between extrinsic environmental and behavioral factors and intrinsic cardiovascular regulatory mechanisms [1]. Although these variations represent a continuous phenomenon, definitions and classification of blood pressure variability patterns have been proposed on the basis of the BP measuring intervals considered for its assessment: beat to beat (**very-short-term** blood pressure variability), within 24 h (minute to minute, hour to hour, and day to night; **short-term** blood pressure variability), over different days (**midterm** blood pressure variability), or over weeks, months, seasons, and years (**long-term** blood pressure variability commonly assessed based on clinic BP values, i.e., as visit-to-visit blood pressure variability) [1]. These different types of blood pressure variability appear to be influenced by several cardiovascular regulatory mechanisms and by subjects' individual characteristics. Their interest comes from the evidence, provided by experimental and observational studies, as well as by their meta-analyses, that an increase in the amplitude of all these types of BP variations is associated with hypertension-mediated organ damage (HMOD) and with an increased risk of cardiovascular events and cardiovascular and all-cause mortality, although we still miss the demonstration by intervention trials that a treatment-induced reduction in blood pressure variability is associated with a better outcome (Fig. 14.1).

The aim of this chapter is to review the available evidence regarding day-by-day home blood pressure variability, its mechanisms, the methodological aspects for its assessment based on home BP measurements as well as its clinical relevance for cardiovascular prognosis. Specific aspects relevant in the light of potential clinical application of home blood pressure variability will also be addressed, such as whether and how it should be assessed in addition to average BP levels, and whether

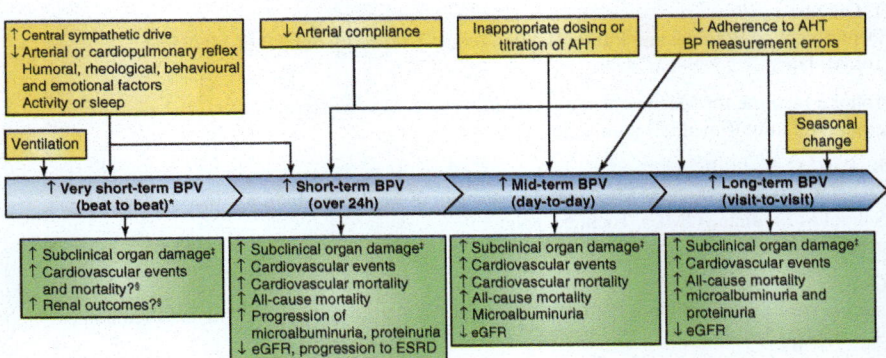

Fig. 14.1 Different types of blood pressure variability, their determinants, and prognostic relevance. Taken from [2] by permission. *Assessed in laboratory conditions; ‡cardiac, vascular, and renal subclinical organ damage; §blood pressure variability on a beat-to-beat basis has not been routinely measured in population studies. Abbreviations: *AHT* antihypertensive treatment, *BP* blood pressure, *BPV* blood pressure variability, *ESRD* end-stage renal disease, *eGFR* estimated glomerular filtration rate

and how antihypertensive treatment strategies should be targeted at reducing not only average BP levels but also the degree of day-by-day blood pressure variability in order to optimize cardiovascular protection. In view of the considerable semantic confusion in the field, in this chapter we will use the term home blood pressure variability in relation to blood pressure variability assessed on a day-to-day basis with self BP monitoring at home. In most cases this is equivalent to day-to-day blood pressure variability or midterm blood pressure variability, although there might be some exceptions (e.g., day-to-day variability of office BP or long-term variability of home BP).

14.2 Factors Associated with Increased Home BPV

When considering midterm blood pressure variability, behavioral factors such as job strain, levels of physical activity, sleep/wakefulness cycles, quality and duration of sleep, postural changes, and patterns of sodium intake have been shown to play an important role in determining the degree of day-by-day BP fluctuations (see Fig. 14.1 and Box 14.1). This is exemplified by studies in which significant changes in BP levels between working days and the weekend have been reported [3]. Population studies have identified several factors associated with increased values of day-by-day blood pressure variability in home measurements such as advanced age, female gender, increased arterial stiffness, elevated mean BP values, low body mass index, low heart

---

Box 14.1: Mechanisms and Factors Responsible for Midterm Blood Pressure Variability

Behavioral factors

- Job strain/home stress
- Levels of physical activity
- Changes of sleep/wakefulness cycles
- Quality and duration of sleep
- Postural changes
- Level of sodium intake
- Smoking/alcohol

Antihypertensive treatment-related factors

- Inconsistent BP control
- Poor patient's adherence to prescribed drugs
- Improper dosing/titration of antihypertensive drugs
- Dose omission or delay in drug intake

Incorrect home BP monitoring conditions

Environmental factors

- Seasonal changes in ambient temperature
- Changes in barometric pressure and altitude above sea level

rate, high heart rate variability, excessive alcohol intake, cigarette smoking, history of peripheral artery disease, cardiovascular disease, diabetes mellitus, diabetic nephropathy, and sedentary lifestyle [4–9]. Of note, a population study in elderly subjects showed higher values of midterm blood pressure variability among subjects with masked and sustained hypertension compared to those with sustained normotension and white-coat hypertension [10]. This study has also suggested that increasing degrees of day-by-day BP fluctuations might prevent the identification of sustained hypertension.

Studies focusing on treated hypertensive patients have found a higher day-by-day blood pressure variability among these individuals compared to untreated subjects [5, 7], also reporting higher values of home blood pressure variability in case of treatment with beta-blockers, short duration of treatment [11], and increasing number of antihypertensive drugs [8].

14.3 Methodological Aspects in the Assessment of Midterm Blood Pressure Variability

Adequate implementation of a proper BP monitoring method, according to current hypertension guidelines recommendations, is critical to guarantee an accurate estimation of BP values and hence of blood pressure variability indices, either for research purposes or in a clinical setting [12–16] (Box 14.2).

The common approach for the evaluation of day-by-day blood pressure variability consists in its assessment from self BP measurements performed by patients at home over several days according to the current ESH recommendations [13, 16, 17]. Although HBPM cannot currently provide information on nighttime BP (except with few novel home BP monitors) nor on 24 h BP profiles (as ABPM does), it is widely available, it has rather low-cost, and is well accepted by patients, while providing adequate BP measures for estimation of day-by-day blood pressure variability, devoid of the white coat effect. Overall, HBPM schedule should consist of duplicate morning and evening BP measurements with validated devices for a 7-day period (at least 3 days required) before each office visit [16]. A recent report of the International Database of Home Blood Pressure in Relation to Cardiovascular Outcome (IDHOCO) study, based on analysis of morning HBP measurements, has indicated that indices of home blood pressure variability may retain their prognostic value even when calculated from a 3-day schedule as compared to the suggested 7-day [18]. Regarding the question on whether morning or evening HBP measures should be considered, evidence from outcome studies is in part controversial, with some studies indicating the superior prognostic value of day-by-day home blood pressure variability determined on the basis of morning BP measures as compared to morning-evening or evening home blood pressure variability [19, 20], while other studies (e.g., the HOMED-BP study) showed evening HBPV before treatment to be a better predictor of outcome [21].

Although the large heterogeneity among studies in terms of measurement schedules (number of readings, number of days, morning and/or evening), BP devices and blood pressure variability indices has not yet allowed to identify the ideal approach for assessment of midterm blood pressure variability based on HBPM [22], some recommendations based on available evidence are presented in Box 14.2.

Box 14.2: Methods of Day-by-Day Blood Pressure Variability Assessment
BP blood pressure, *BPV* blood pressure variations, *ABPM* ambulatory blood pressure monitoring, *HBPM* home blood pressure monitoring, *OBP* office blood pressure, *SD* standard deviation, *CV* coefficient of variation, *ARV* average real variability, *VIM* variability independent of the mean

- **Devices:** Use of validated automated oscillometric upper-arm cuff devices
- **Method for BP measurement:** HBPM
- **Measurement intervals:**
  - Day-by-day
  - From morning to evening
- **Number of measurements:** For HBPM duplicate BP measurements (1 min apart) in the morning and in the evening for each day
- **Time of measurement:**
  - Morning and evening before food and/or drug intake (some guidelines recommend only morning readings)
  - Perform HBPM during usual working days
- **Time of measurement in treated patients:** Morning and evening BP measurements before drug intake (patients should be under stable treatment)
- **Duration of the recording period and measurement sequence:**
  - HBP measurement schedule over several (preferably 7 and at least 3) working days is suggested as the optimal approach before each office visit, with this sequence repeated after weeks or months when assessing the effects of treatment
  - Duplicate morning and evening measurements, taken at 1-min interval after a 5-min rest (for the comparative assessment of morning vs. evening vs. morning-evening combination)
- **Editing.** No editing is recommended at present (apart from discarding first day measurements)
- **Main indices of blood pressure variability:** SD, CV, ARV, VIM, morning-evening changes, maximum-minimum values
- **Advantages** inexpensive, well accepted by patients.
- **Possible disadvantages**
  - Patients' training required for HBPM
  - Possibility of measurements in selected conditions only and misreporting of readings
  - Data for blood pressure variability calculation must be entered manually, unless devices with data storage and transfer capabilities are used

14.3.1 Indices for Assessment of Midterm Blood Pressure Variability

Changes occurring in home BP values obtained over a number of days may be estimated by applying several indices that may be grouped into three main categories: indices of dispersion of BP values, indices reflecting their sequential changes, and indices estimating BP instability (Table 14.1).

Standard deviation (SD) represents the most traditional and commonly used index for assessment of blood pressure variability and provides a measure of values dispersion over selected time windows [23, 24]. Since SD increases with increasing average BP values, **the coefficient of variation (CV)** may be applied [23] in order to account for this dependence. **Average Real Variability (ARV)** is an index of overall variability based on readings sequence. It is computed as the average of the absolute differences between consecutive BP measurements. It focuses on the sequence of BP readings, thus reflecting reading-to-reading, within-subject variability in BP values [25]. When considering ambulatory BP recordings over the 24 h, ARV has been shown to be a more specific estimate of BP variability and a more effective predictor of outcome than conventional SD [12, 25, 26]. Like SD, ARV is correlated with mean BP levels, but at variance from the former, it effectively removes the contribution of trends in mean BP to overall blood pressure variability. Other indices of variability based on reading sequence include **time rate of BP variation** (similar to ARV but quantified as a function of time to provide information also on speed of BP changes) and **interval weighted SD** (similar to SD), both of which take into account the interval between measurements giving larger weight to more distant pairs of readings. **Variability Independent of the Mean (VIM)** excludes the effect of mean BP on blood pressure variability by applying non-linear

Table 14.1 Indices for estimation of midterm blood pressure variability

Type of index	Index	Formula
Dispersion	Standard deviation (SD)	$SD = \sqrt{\dfrac{1}{N-1}\sum_{i=1}^{N}\left(BP_i - \overline{BP}\right)^2}$
	Coefficient of variation (CV)	$CV = 100 * SD / \overline{BP}$
	Variability independent of the mean (VIM)	$VIM = \dfrac{SD}{\overline{BP}^x} * \overline{BP_P}^x$
Sequence	Average real variability (ARV)	$ARV = \dfrac{1}{N-1}\sum_{i=1}^{N-1}\left|BP_{i+1} - BP_i\right|$
	Interval weighted SD (wSD)	$iSD = \sqrt{\dfrac{1}{\sum W_i}\sum_{i=1}^{N}W_i\left(BP_i - \overline{BP}\right)^2}$
	Time rate of BP variation	$TR = \dfrac{\sum_{i=1}^{N-1}|r_i|}{N-1}$
Instability	Range (maximum–minimum BP)	Range = Max − Min
	Peak size (maximum BP)	Peak = Max − mean
	Trough size (mean-minimum BP)	Trough = Mean − Min

regression analysis (i.e., plotting SD against mean) [27]. For its estimation, it requires calculation of a factor x from overall population data. Midterm blood pressure variability may also be assessed by applying **Instability indices** which take into account extreme readings of the distribution of BP values within a given time window such as **Range (maximum-minimum BP), Peak size (maximum BP), and Trough size (mean-minimum BP)**. These indices appear to have different strengths and limitations. Although some studies have demonstrated their clinical value, a major limitation of these indices is that extreme readings have a limited reliability within a given distribution of values, especially when focusing on individual subjects, being unstable and prone to show measurement artifacts more than actual BP values. Until data showing the superiority of one or more of these indices become available, it is difficult to yield any recommendation on which among them should be selected.

14.4   Clinical Relevance of Midterm Blood Pressure Variability

The clinical relevance of midterm blood pressure variability has been supported by the evidence accumulated in last decades showing its predictive value for target-organ damage and cardiovascular morbidity and mortality outcomes. Overall, the studies addressing the predictive value of midterm blood pressure variability for HMOD have been characterized by significant heterogeneity in the methodology for evaluating blood pressure variability (home BP monitoring schedule, variability indices, characteristics of subjects) and by discrepant results regarding impact on outcome [22]. Overall, it seems that there is not a single index of blood pressure variability nor an index of target-organ damage with consistent and independent relationships with midterm blood pressure variability that might be found systematically in all the positive and negative studies available [22, 28–35].

Regarding cardiovascular events, the most solid evidence supporting the prognostic value of midterm blood pressure variability is derived from the IDHOCO database, composed of 4 populations ($n = 6.238$, 22% treated hypertensive subjects) [18]. An analysis of this database based on day-to-day morning home BP measurements showed all indices of systolic/diastolic blood pressure variability (SD, CV, ARV, VIM) to be independently associated with all-cause and cardiovascular mortality [18]. However, regarding the question on whether midterm blood pressure variability may independently add to cardiovascular risk stratification, the IDHOCO analysis revealed only a minor-nonsignificant incremental improvement for home blood pressure variability in terms of net reclassification and integrated discrimination improvements, a conclusion, however, which might have been partly undermined by the heterogeneity of the methodologies adopted in the studies considered [18]. A recent meta-analysis of observational cohorts and of clinical trials by Stevens et al. reported significant hazard ratios for cardiovascular events as well as for cardiovascular and all-cause mortality in relation to an increased midterm blood pressure variability after accounting for confounders [36]. Although a direct head-to-head comparison between all types of blood pressure variability in terms of prognosis has not been addressed so far, it is important to note that the meta-analysis by Stevens et al. showed similar hazard ratios for all-cause mortality among all types of systolic blood pressure variability [long term (Visit-to-visit): 1.12 (95% confidence intervals: 1.05, 1.20); midterm (day-by-day home): 1.15 (1.06, 1.26); short term (24-h ambulatory): 1.11 (1.04. 1.18)] [36]. In addition, it appears that morning day-by-day home blood pressure variability has the strongest prognostic value as compared to morning-evening or evening home blood pressure variability [19, 37]. Of note, this meta-analysis reported standardized hazard ratios to account for the heterogeneity in reporting of risk per different units across studies [36] (Fig. 14.2).

Recently, the independent predictive value of measures of home blood pressure variability was confirmed by a report of the Didima study, aimed at comparatively exploring the prognostic value of home BP average and variability versus office BP measurements over a 19-year follow-up. Although both office BP and HBP variability predicted total mortality and cardiovascular risk, indices of systolic HBP variability showed a superior prognostic value for incident total mortality and cardiovascular events than measures of variability obtained from office BP measures [38].

A recent report of the J-HOP Study (Japan Morning Surge-Home Blood Pressure) evaluated the relationship between day-by-day home blood pressure variability (as assessed through VIM) and incident cardiovascular events (including coronary heart disease and stroke) in a large sample of 4231 subjects from Japan. After a 4-year follow-up period (16750.3 person-years), VIMSBP was associated with cardiovascular disease risk (hazard ratio per 1-SD increase, 1.32; 95% confidence interval [CI], 1.15–1.52), independently of mean home SBP levels. Adding VIMSBP to different cardiovascular disease prediction models significantly improved discrimination and reclassification of subjects (C statistic, 0.785 versus 0.770; C statistic difference, 0.015; 95% CI, 0.003–0.028). These findings suggest that assessment of home SBP variability, in addition to average home SBP levels, may improve risk of cardiovascular disease prediction and helps in discrimination between high- and low-risk groups among Japanese outpatients [39].

Regarding potential threshold values for midterm blood pressure variability, the IDHOCO study provided some relevant evidence indicating that the risk of cardiovascular morbidity and mortality was steeply increased in the highest decile of systolic/diastolic home blood pressure variability (CV $\geq 11/12.8\%$, respectively) [18]. These data need however to be validated by other studies.

Finally, whether antihypertensive treatment strategies should be targeted at reducing not only average BP levels but also the degree of day-by-day HBPV in order to optimize cardiovascular protection is still an open question. A study by Matsui et al. evaluating the response of midterm blood pressure variability to antihypertensive treatment showed that, compared to olmesartan/hydrochlorothiazide combination, the combination of olmesartan/azelnidipine improved home blood pressure variability (home BP monitoring was performed before each office visit for a total of 7 visits during a 24-week period) in addition to average home BP reduction, and that the reduction in home blood pressure variability was associated with the reduction in arterial stiffness in the group randomized to azelnidipine [33]. On the contrary, in a study conducted in 310 hypertensive subjects, the treatment-induced reduction in urine albumin excretion after a 6-month period of antihypertensive treatment with candesartan (+diuretics) was significantly associated with a

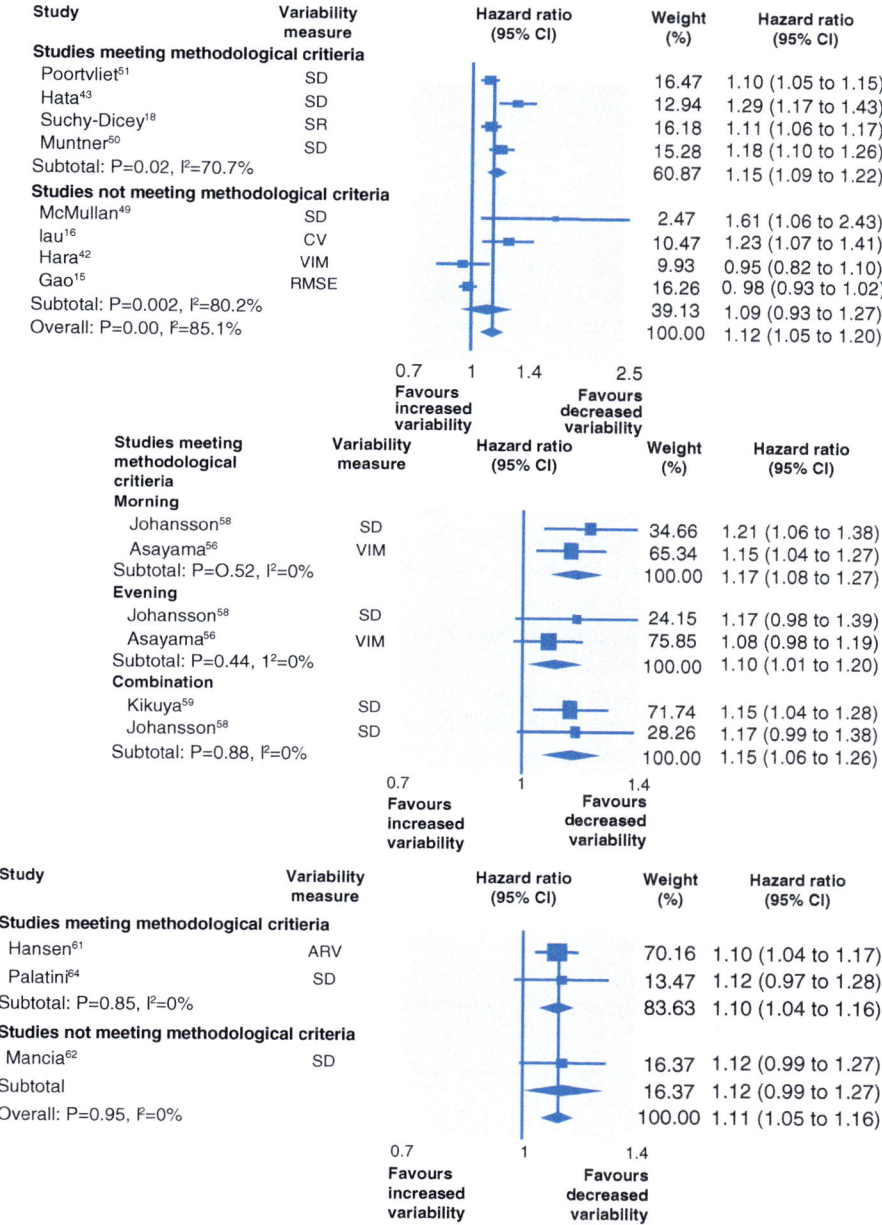

Fig. 14.2 Hazard ratios for all-cause mortality for increases in clinic systolic blood pressure variability (upper panel); in home systolic blood pressure variability (middle panel) or in ambulatory systolic blood pressure variability (lower panel). Modified from Stevens et al. [36] by permission

reduction in average home BP but was not associated with a reduction in the SD of home SBP or in the maximum home SBP [40]. In the same line, a report of the (Hypertension Objective treatment based on Measurement by Electrical Devices of BP) study did not find any significant impact of antihypertensive drug classes on blood pressure variability changes [21].

14.5   Conclusions

Although evidence from some recent studies has indicated an incremental contribution of blood pressure variability for cardiovascular risk stratification, over and above the impact of average BP values, the relevance of such contribution has been shown to be influenced by the methodology employed for assessment of blood pressure variability and by the characteristics and baseline cardiovascular risk of the study populations. Future studies should establish whether there are specific categories of patients (high versus low risk, treated or untreated) where home blood pressure variability might more clearly provide additional predictive information over and above the impact of average BP levels. While many indices of midterm blood pressure variability have been shown to be of prognostic value, no interventional longitudinal outcome study has yet been conducted specifically addressing which is the best index of midterm blood pressure variability that could provide protection when reduced by treatment, thus offering indications for clinical practice. Although some outcome studies addressing the prognostic value of blood pressure variability have suggested reference values and thresholds for blood pressure variability, the heterogeneity in the indices of blood pressure variability used and the different characteristics of study populations have not allowed to definitely conclude on what midterm blood pressure variability levels should be regarded as normal [22]. Similarly, although a series of studies and *post hoc* analyses of clinical trials in hypertension have addressed whether there are drugs able to specifically reduce blood pressure variability and whether such reduction is translated into an improved cardiovascular risk, no intervention study has yet formally explored this issue. Thus, home blood pressure variability should at present still be seen as a research issue, while waiting for the results of ongoing clinical trials on its actual prognostic relevance.

References

1. Parati G, Ochoa JE, Lombardi C, Bilo G. Assessment and management of blood-pressure variability. Nat Rev Cardiol. 2013;10(3):143–55.
2. Parati G, Ochoa JE, Bilo G. Blood pressure variability, cardiovascular risk, and risk for renal disease progression. Curr Hypertens Rep. 2012;14(5):421–31.
3. Murakami S, Otsuka K, Kubo Y, Shinagawa M, Matsuoka O, Yamanaka T, et al. Weekly variation of home and ambulatory blood pressure and relation between arterial stiffness and blood pressure measurements in community-dwelling hypertensives. Clin Exp Hypertens. 2005;27:231–9.
4. Niiranen TJ, Hanninen MR, Johansson J, Reunanen A, Jula AM. Home-measured blood pressure is a stronger predictor of cardiovascular risk than office blood pressure: the Finn-Home study. Hypertension. 2010;55(6):1346–51.

5. Thijs L, Staessen JA, Celis H, Fagard R, De Cort P, de Gaudemaris R, et al. The international database of self-recorded blood pressures in normotensive and untreated hypertensive subjects. Blood Press Monit. 1999;4(2):77–86.
6. Nagai M, Hoshide S, Ishikawa J, Shimada K, Kario K. Visit-to-visit blood pressure variations: new independent determinants for carotid artery measures in the elderly at high risk of cardiovascular disease. J Am Soc Hypertens. 2011;5(3):184–92.
7. Niiranen TJ, Asayama K, Thijs L, Johansson JK, Ohkubo T, Kikuya M, et al. Outcome-driven thresholds for home blood pressure measurement: international database of home blood pressure in relation to cardiovascular outcome. Hypertension. 2013;61(1):27–34.
8. Okada T, Nakao T, Matsumoto H, Nagaoka Y, Tomaru R, Iwasawa H, et al. Day-by-day variability of home blood pressure in patients with chronic kidney disease. Nihon Jinzo Gakkai shi. 2008;50(5):588–96.
9. Kato T, Kikuya M, Ohkubo T, Satoh M, Hara A, Obara T, et al. Factors associated with day-by-day variability of self-measured blood pressure at home: the Ohasama study. Am J Hypertens. 2010;23(9):980–6.
10. Cacciolati C, Tzourio C, Hanon O. Blood pressure variability in elderly persons with white-coat and masked hypertension compared to those with normotension and sustained hypertension. Am J Hypertens. 2013;26(3):367–72.
11. Ishikura K, Obara T, Kato T, Kikuya M, Shibamiya T, Shinki T, et al. Associations between day-by-day variability in blood pressure measured at home and antihypertensive drugs: the J-HOME-morning study. Clin Exp Hypertens. 2012;34(4):297–304.
12. O'Brien E, Parati G, Stergiou G, Asmar R, Beilin L, Bilo G, et al. European Society of Hypertension position paper on ambulatory blood pressure monitoring. J Hypertens. 2013;31(9):1731–68.
13. Williams B, Mancia G, Spiering W, Agabiti Rosei E, Azizi M, Burnier M, et al. 2018 practice guidelines for the management of arterial hypertension of the European Society of Hypertension and the European Society of Cardiology: ESH/ESC task force for the Management of Arterial Hypertension. J Hypertens. 2018;36(12):2284–309.
14. Parati G, Stergiou G, O'Brien E, Asmar R, Beilin L, Bilo G, et al. European Society of Hypertension practice guidelines for ambulatory blood pressure monitoring. J Hypertens. 2014;32(7):1359–66.
15. Stergiou GS, Parati G, Vlachopoulos C, Achimastos A, Andreadis E, Asmar R, et al. Methodology and technology for peripheral and central blood pressure and blood pressure variability measurement: current status and future directions - position statement of the European Society of Hypertension Working Group on blood pressure monitoring and cardiovascular variability. J Hypertens. 2016;34(9):1665–77.
16. Parati G, Stergiou GS, Asmar R, Bilo G, de Leeuw P, Imai Y, et al. European Society of Hypertension guidelines for blood pressure monitoring at home: a summary report of the second international consensus conference on home blood pressure monitoring. J Hypertens. 2008;26(8):1505–26.
17. Stergiou GS, Parati G, McManus RJ, Head GA, Myers MG, Whelton PK. Guidelines for blood pressure measurement: development over 30 years. J Clin Hypertens (Greenwich). 2018;20(7):1089–91.
18. Juhanoja EP, Niiranen TJ, Johansson JK, Puukka PJ, Thijs L, Asayama K, et al. Outcome-driven thresholds for increased home blood pressure variability. Hypertension. 2017;69(4):599–607.
19. Johansson JK, Niiranen TJ, Puukka PJ, Jula AM. Prognostic value of the variability in home-measured blood pressure and heart rate: the Finn-home study. Hypertension. 2012;59(2):212–8.
20. Asayama K, Kikuya M, Schutte R, Thijs L, Hosaka M, Satoh M, et al. Home blood pressure variability as cardiovascular risk factor in the population of Ohasama. Hypertension. 2013;61(1):61–9.
21. Asayama K, Ohkubo T, Hanazawa T, Watabe D, Hosaka M, Satoh M, et al. Does antihypertensive drug class affect day-to-day variability of self-measured home blood pressure? The HOMED-BP study. J Am Heart Assoc. 2016;5(3):e002995.
22. Stergiou GS, Ntineri A, Kollias A, Ohkubo T, Imai Y, Parati G. Blood pressure variability assessed by home measurements: a systematic review. Hypertens Res. 2014;37(6):565–72.

23. di Rienzo M, Grassi G, Pedotti A, Mancia G. Continuous vs intermittent blood pressure measurements in estimating 24-hour average blood pressure. Hypertension. 1983;5(2):264–9.
24. Mancia G, Di Rienzo M, Parati G. Ambulatory blood pressure monitoring use in hypertension research and clinical practice. Hypertension. 1993;21(4):510–24.
25. Mena L, Pintos S, Queipo NV, Aizpurua JA, Maestre G, Sulbaran T. A reliable index for the prognostic significance of blood pressure variability. J Hypertens. 2005;23(3):505–11.
26. Hansen TW, Thijs L, Li Y, Boggia J, Kikuya M, Bjorklund-Bodegard K, et al. Prognostic value of reading-to-reading blood pressure variability over 24 hours in 8938 subjects from 11 populations. Hypertension. 2010;55(4):1049–57.
27. Rothwell PM, Howard SC, Dolan E, O'Brien E, Dobson JE, Dahlof B, et al. Prognostic significance of visit-to-visit variability, maximum systolic blood pressure, and episodic hypertension. Lancet. 2010;375(9718):895–905.
28. Veloudi P, Blizzard CL, Head GA, Abhayaratna WP, Stowasser M, Sharman JE. Blood pressure variability and prediction of target organ damage in patients with uncomplicated hypertension. Am J Hypertens. 2016;29(9):1046–54.
29. Wei FF, Li Y, Zhang L, Xu TY, Ding FH, Wang JG, et al. Beat-to-beat, reading-to-reading, and day-to-day blood pressure variability in relation to organ damage in untreated Chinese. Hypertension. 2014;63(4):790–6.
30. Shibasaki S, Hoshide S, Eguchi K, Ishikawa J, Kario K. Japan morning surge-home blood pressure study G. Increase trend in home blood pressure on a single occasion is associated with B-type natriuretic peptide and the estimated glomerular filtration rate. Am J Hypertens. 2015;28(9):1098–105.
31. Ushigome E, Fukui M, Hamaguchi M, Tanaka T, Atsuta H, Mogami S, et al. Maximum home systolic blood pressure is a useful indicator of arterial stiffness in patients with type 2 diabetes mellitus: post hoc analysis of a cross-sectional multicenter study. Diabetes Res Clin Pract. 2014;105(3):344–51.
32. Liu Z, Zhao Y, Lu F, Zhang H, Diao Y. Day-by-day variability in self-measured blood pressure at home: effects on carotid artery atherosclerosis, brachial flow-mediated dilation, and endothelin-1 in normotensive and mild-moderate hypertensive individuals. Blood Press Monit. 2013;18(6):316–25.
33. Matsui Y, O'Rourke MF, Hoshide S, Ishikawa J, Shimada K, Kario K. Combined effect of angiotensin II receptor blocker and either a calcium channel blocker or diuretic on day-by-day variability of home blood pressure: the Japan combined treatment with Olmesartan and a Calcium-Channel blocker versus Olmesartan and diuretics randomized efficacy study. Hypertension. 2012;59(6):1132–8.
34. Ushigome E, Fukui M, Hamaguchi M, Senmaru T, Sakabe K, Tanaka M, et al. The coefficient variation of home blood pressure is a novel factor associated with macroalbuminuria in type 2 diabetes mellitus. Hypertens Res. 2011;34(12):1271–5.
35. Matsui Y, Ishikawa J, Eguchi K, Shibasaki S, Shimada K, Kario K. Maximum value of home blood pressure: a novel indicator of target organ damage in hypertension. Hypertension. 2011;57(6):1087–93.
36. Stevens SL, Wood S, Koshiaris C, Law K, Glasziou P, Stevens RJ, et al. Blood pressure variability and cardiovascular disease: systematic review and meta-analysis. BMJ. 2016;354:i4098.
37. Ohkubo T, Asayama K, Kikuya M, Metoki H, Hoshi H, Hashimoto J, et al. How many times should blood pressure be measured at home for better prediction of stroke risk? Ten-year follow-up results from the Ohasama study. J Hypertens. 2004;22(6):1099–104.
38. Ntineri A, Kalogeropoulos PG, Kyriakoulis KG, Aissopou EK, Thomopoulou G, Kollias A, et al. Prognostic value of average home blood pressure and variability: 19-year follow-up of the Didima study. J Hypertens. 2018;36(1):69–76.
39. Hoshide S, Yano Y, Mizuno H, Kanegae H, Kario K. Day-by-day variability of home blood pressure and incident cardiovascular disease in clinical practice: the J-HOP study (Japan morning surge-home blood pressure). Hypertension. 2018;71(1):177–84.
40. Hoshide S, Yano Y, Shimizu M, Eguchi K, Ishikawa J, Kario K. Is home blood pressure variability itself an interventional target beyond lowering mean home blood pressure during antihypertensive treatment? Hypertens Res. 2012;35(8):862–6.

Home Versus Ambulatory Blood Pressure Monitoring

15

Eoin O'Brien, Alex de la Sierra, Richard J. McManus,
Anastasia Mihailidou, Paul Muntner, Martin G. Myers,
George S. Stergiou, Gianfranco Parati, and Efstathios Manios

E. O'Brien (✉)
The Conway Institute, University College Dublin, Dublin, Ireland

A. de la Sierra
Department of Internal Medicine, Hospital Mutua Terrassa, University of Barcelona,
Barcelona, Catalonia, Spain
e-mail: adelasierra@mutuaterrassa.cat

R. J. McManus
Nuffield Department of Primary Care Health Sciences,
University of Oxford, Radcliffe Observatory Quarter, Oxford, UK
e-mail: richard.mcmanus@phc.ox.ac.uk

A. Mihailidou
Cardiovascular & Hormonal Research Laboratory, Department of Cardiology and Kolling
Institute, Royal North Shore Hospital, St Leonards, NSW, Australia

Macquarie University, Sydney, NSW, Australia
e-mail: anastasia.mihailidou@health.nsw.gov.au

P. Muntner
Department of Epidemiology, University of Alabama at Birmingham, Birmingham, AL, USA
e-mail: pmuntner@uab.edu

M. G. Myers
Department of Cardiology, Schulich Heart Program, Sunnybrook Health Sciences Centre,
Toronto, ON, Canada

Department of Medicine, University of Toronto, Toronto, ON, Canada
e-mail: martin.myers@sunnybrook.ca

G. S. Stergiou
Hypertension Center STRIDE-7, National and Kapodistrian University of Athens, School of
Medicine, Third Department of Medicine, Sotiria Hospital, Athens, Greece
e-mail: gstergi@med.uoa.gr

G. Parati
Department of Medicine and Surgery, University of Milano-Bicocca, Milan, Italy

Istituto Auxologico Italiano, IRCCS, Department of Cardiovascular, Neural and Metabolic
Sciences, Milan, Italy
e-mail: gianfranco.parati@unimib.it

E. Manios
Department of Clinical Therapeutics, National and Kapodistrian University of Athens,
Medical School, Alexandra Hospital, Athens, Greece

15.1   Introduction

While office BP measurement (OBPM) remains commonly used, in recent years it has been largely superseded for treatment initiation and titration by out-of-office measurement. Although in the past OBPM was used to guide the decision to initiate and titrate therapy, it is now generally accepted that it should be used only as a screening technique, with out-of-office measurements being required in most cases before diagnostic or therapeutic decisions are made [1–8]. The rationale for this recommendation is based on the fact that OBPM is subject to two major environmental influences that make it unrepresentative of the true BP, namely the white-coat response (giving misleadingly high office measurements in the face of a normal mean out-of-office BP) and masked hypertension (giving misleadingly low office readings in the face of hypertensive out-of-office BP) [3].

Although ABPM has been available for over 40 years, it has only recently been accepted as the most reliable and accurate measurement of BP [8], which has led international guidelines to focus more on the use of ABPM for diagnosing hypertension. However, recent guidelines are now giving greater attention to a wider role for ABPM in assessing the response to therapy and additional information that may be provided by identifying specific patterns of BP behaviour [3, 6, 8].

Although HBPM does not give as much information as ABPM, it is widely available, relatively inexpensive and well accepted by patients. Consequently, current guidelines recommend HBPM as an essential method for the evaluation of BP in untreated subjects with suspected hypertension and for monitoring BP control in treated hypertensive patients [7].

15.2   Ambulatory Blood Pressure Measurement (ABPM)

15.2.1 Advantages of ABPM

ABPM can provide information that assists in the diagnosis and management of patients with hypertension, over and above the information derived from other forms of measurement:

Diagnosis of white-coat and masked hypertension: International and national guidelines, having carefully examined the evidence as to which method of BP measurement is best—office, home or ABPM—have unanimously recommended ABPM as the 'gold standard' technology for BP measurement [3]. The rationale behind these recommendations is to confirm that the elevation of BP noted with conventional office measurement is sustained and not due to a white-coat reaction, as may occur in some 25% of subjects, and to identify patients with masked hypertension [9].

White-coat hypertension may be diagnosed from ABPM if BP elevation during the first hour of measurement is present and, in the absence of an office BP, provides a means of diagnosing the white-coat phenomenon [10]. Likewise, white-coat effect—elevation of BP in the first hour of recording that is higher than daytime BP, may also be evident on ABPM. [11] It is more difficult to diagnose masked hypertension than white-coat hypertension, simply because greater discretion is needed to determine which patients with a normal office BP should have ABPM, but the identification of the condition is very important because patients with masked hypertension are at high risk [12]. ABPM has been shown to be superior to HBPM in identifying patients with masked hypertension. The use of ABPM for diagnosing masked hypertension should be guided by suspecting the condition in certain patients. For example, masked hypertension should be suspected in patients with normal (and especially high normal) office BP who have had a previous cardiovascular event (any evidence of cerebrovascular, coronary, vascular, or renovascular disease), patients with concomitant disease (diabetes, metabolic syndrome), and patients with a substantial family history of hypertension or cardiovascular disease [3]. ABPM can also disclose the phenomenon of masked uncontrolled hypertension, a condition in which patients receiving treatment for hypertension have normal office BP but elevated out-of-office BP. Identification of this condition is important because it carries a high risk for cardiovascular events [13].

Detection of patterns of blood pressure behaviour: Abnormal patterns of BP behaviour may indicate specific forms of hypertension, such as nocturnal hypertension, or may be associated with concomitant illnesses, such as sleep apnoea, and recognition of these abnormal patterns of BP behaviour during the daytime and/or the night-time periods can be helpful in the diagnosis and management of hypertension [6, 14–18]. ABPM can also provide an assessment of short-term BP variability over 24 h, which has been shown to carry prognostic information [19, 20]. These patterns of 24-hour BP behaviour are listed in Table 15.1.

There has been a tendency in clinical practice to concentrate on daytime pressures provided by ABPM, as they are thought to be closer to OBPM. However, the association of night-time hypertension with the cardiovascular consequences of hypertension, such as stroke, has focussed the scientific literature on nocturnal hypertensive patterns, such as isolated nocturnal hypertension, and a non-dipping pattern of BP [6, 11, 14–18] (Table 15.1). Indeed, on-going research may show that night-time BP better represents baseline BP measurement, but, at present, it is important to be aware that there may be causes for nocturnal hypertension, such as obstructive sleep apnoea (OSA) [21], and the increased risk of stroke with elevated nocturnal BP, makes it important to assess the response to BP lowering medication during sleep. In some patients, the nocturnal decline in BP may be absent (non-dipping) so that BP does not decrease to at least 10% below daytime BP. In some instances, BP may even rise during sleeping hours to reach levels that are higher than daytime levels (reverse dipping or rising), and these patients are at highest risk. Alternatively, there may be a marked fall in BP during the night window to give the phenomenon of extreme dipping [6, 11, 14]. The magnitude of the rise in BP in the morning—the 'morning surge'—around the time of awakening may also yield additional prognostic information [7, 11].

Diagnosis of hypotension: Treatment may cause excessive lowering of BP, especially in the frail elderly, when avoiding falls and their resultant morbidity becomes extremely important [6, 11, 22]. Recent evidence suggests that some patients may

Table 15.1 Patterns of ambulatory blood pressure [6]

Daytime hypertension	
White-coat hypertension	
White-coat effect	
Systolic and diastolic hypertension	
Isolated systolic hypertension	
Isolated diastolic hypertension	
Siesta dipping/post-prandial hypotension	
Nocturnal hypertension	
Dipping:	Nocturnal BP fall >10% of daytime values or Night/day BP ratio <0.9 and >0.8—normal diurnal BP pattern
*Reduced dipping:**	Nocturnal BP fall from 1 to 10% of daytime values or Night/day BP ratio <1 and >0.9—reduced diurnal BP pattern
Non-dipping & nocturnal risers:	No reduction or increase in nocturnal BP or Night/day ratio ≥1—associated with poor cardiovascular risk
Nocturnal risers:	Nocturnal BP greater than daytime BP
Extreme dipping:	Marked nocturnal BP fall >20% of daytime values or Night/day ratio <0.8—debatable cardiovascular risk
Nocturnal hypertension:	Increased absolute level of night time BP Associated with increased cardiovascular risk—may indicate OSA
Morning surge:	Excessive BP elevation rising in morning Definitions, thresholds and prognostic impact debatable
Short term BP variability	
Quantified as 24 h Standard Deviation (SD) or Coefficient of Variation (CV), 24 h Weighted SD or CV, or Average Real Variability of either SBP and DBP	
[**The classic definition of non-dipping (Nocturnal BP fall <10% or Night/day ratio >0.9) may be criticized because 'reduced dipping' is in effect a form of 'non-dipping']	
Ambulatory hypotension	
Spontaneous, postural, post-prandial and drug-induced hypotensive patterns	

be adversely affected by marked lowering of nocturnal BP [22]. It is important, therefore, to use ABPM to detect an excessive decrease in BP with medication, especially at night. This is especially relevant in the light of the recent US guidelines for hypertension which advocate a target blood pressure below 130/80mmHg for many patients, including the elderly. [8]

15.2.2 Practical Considerations

Frequency of ABPM: ABPM is beneficial in guiding drug prescribing by identifying patients who need more antihypertensive therapy. In patients with a low risk profile, ABPM might be repeated every few months until control is achieved. If the cardiovascular risk of the patient is high (evidence of target organ damage, previous cardiovascular event, bad family history, or comorbidities, such as diabetes), the need to achieve good BP control becomes more pressing. So once treatment is initiated, it would seem reasonable to repeat ABPM within a few weeks to determine whether adequate reduction has been achieved, but as some individuals will not tolerate frequent ABPM, HBPM is a useful alternative to reduce the need for repeated ABPM [6, 11].

Devices that detect both ABPM and atrial fibrillation (AF): In the elderly, AF now constitutes a mini-epidemic within the larger epidemic of hypertension affecting older age-groups. Given the potential benefits of detecting asymptomatic AF, devices that can combine ABPM with AF detection should be the choice for elderly hypertensive in clinical practice, and manufacturers should be encouraged not only to develop such devices, but to have them validated and evaluated according to internationally accepted standards [23].

15.3   Home Blood Pressure Measurement (HBPM)

15.3.1 Advantages of HBPM

Although HBPM is not as informative as ABPM, the technique provides information that is superior to OBPM and complimentary to ABPM [4, 24]. HBPM provides multiple BP measurements for days, weeks or months away from the artificial office setting and in the usual environment of each individual, thereby allowing thereby a more accurate and representative assessment than with OBPM. HBPM is performed seated at home under relatively stable conditions whereas ABPM is subject to movement, changes in posture and sleep [25, 26]. HBPM allows the detection of white-coat and masked hypertension and is superior to the conventional OBPM in predicting cardiovascular events. HBPM predicts cardiovascular mortality and cardiovascular events after adjusting for OBPM and allows more accurate risk stratification, particularly in patients with masked hypertension [4, 27, 28]. HBPM also allows the assessment of day by day BP variability, which may contribute to outcome prediction [29].

Availability and acceptance by patients: HBPM is widely available in many countries and well accepted by patients [4, 26–28]. Patients prefer HBPM rather than ABPM, particularly for repeated long-term use, as it causes less discomfort and restriction of daily activities and sleep [29]. HBPM increases awareness and patients are motivated to become actively involved in improving BP control [4].

Treatment adjustment: Treated hypertensives who perform HBPM achieve better BP control rates due to improved long-term adherence to drug therapy [30]. Treatment adjustment based on HBPM has been shown to reduce the risk of cardiovascular events [31–33].

The main advantages and differences of HBPM in comparison to office and ambulatory BP are presented in Table 15.2.

Table 15.2 Comparison of the features of office, ambulatory and home blood pressure measurements [4]

Feature	Office	Ambulatory	Home
Detection of white-coat hypertension	−	++	++
Detection of masked hypertension	−	++	++
Assessment of night-time BP level and dip	−	++	+
Assessment of morning BP surge	−	++	−
Assessment of morning hypertension	+/−	++	++
Assessment of antihypertensive drug action	+	++	++
Assessment of duration of drug action	+/−	++	+
Long-term follow-up of hypertension	++	+/−	++
Improvement of patients' compliance	+	−	++
Improvement of hypertension control rate	+	−	++
Reproducibility	−	++	++
Prognostic value	+	++	++
Availability	++	−	++
Cost	−	−	++

15.3.2 Practical Considerations

Devices: Advancement in the technology of HBPM devices has extended their application in clinical practice. Newer automated HBPM devices are capable of screening for AF during routine BP measurement in the elderly with considerable diagnostic accuracy [23, 34]. In addition, HBPM devices are being developed that can provide automated monitoring during night-time sleep to evaluate nocturnal hypertension and to identify non-dippers [4, 18].

Unbiased reporting of HBPM readings by storing values in a device's memory should be encouraged to avoid over- or under-reporting of self-measurements [24, 32, 33, 35]. Reporting bias can be avoided by using home monitors which have automated storage of all BP readings for verification by trained staff, or mobile link, or PC download or with tele-monitoring techniques [4, 25, 26]. Patients should also be asked to record their HBPM readings on a form according to the recommended monitoring schedule.

Monitoring schedule: Current European and US guidelines recommend a standard 7-day HBPM schedule for the initial evaluation of an untreated patient's BP status, after any change in antihypertensive treatment regimen, and also before routine visits to the doctor (for treated hypertensives). This should include duplicate measurements (with 1-min interval) in the morning (before drug intake if treated), and in the evening, for 7 days (at least 4 days). Readings from the first HBPM day should better be discarded, as they might be higher and more variable than of the next days. Thus, HBPM for 4–7 days and then exclusion of the first day (leaving 12–28 readings) should be averaged to give values for decision-making. However, this regimen may prove arduous for some patients. For the long-term follow-up of treated hypertensives, HBPM once or twice per week or less frequently may be sufficient to ensure maintenance of adequate BP control [4, 25, 26].

Thresholds: Several cross-sectional studies have shown considerable diagnostic agreement between HBPM and ABPM, with similar normalcy thresholds, reproducibility, diagnostic accuracy for white-coat and masked hypertension, and prognostic value, with all these features being superior to those of conventional OBP measurements. However, outcome studies have shown that the two methods are not fully interchangeable, and ABPM and HBPM should be regarded as complementary rather than competitive in the assessment of an elevated BP [4, 25]. This issue is highlighted by the differences between ABPM and HBPM in identifying patents with masked hypertension [12].

15.4 Conclusion

There has been a remarkable shift in emphasis in the last decade from inaccurate methods of BP measurement, such as routine manual OBPM, to out-of-office technologies, such as HBPM and ABPM. The diagnosis of hypertension should be made using ABPM, or HBPM if ABPM is not available or not tolerated. Response to drug therapy should be determined by ABPM, or HBPM. If OBPM measurement is used, it should be standardised by utilising automated oscillometric sphygmomanometers preferably with the patients alone to avoid a white-coat effect. Manufacturers of BP measuring devices must now be persuaded to provide inexpensive accurate devices for ABPM and HBPM, which have been validated using established standards. Indeed, technology is now at such an advanced level that it should be possible to provide a single reasonably priced device capable of measuring BP in the office, at home or over 24 h, as required, thereby allowing measurement according to circumstance with one device that would categorise BP measurement according to circumstance rather than methodology—in effect, 'a device for all seasons'.

Acknowledgment *Conflict of Interest*: EOB, GP, and GS have conducted validation studies for various manufacturers and advised manufacturers on device development. ASM—has advised manufacturers on device development. EM—no conflict of interest. RM—has received BP monitors for research from Omron.

References

1. O'Brien E, Dolan E, Stergiou GS. Achieving reliable blood pressure measurements in clinical practice: It's time to meet the challenge. J Clin Hypertens (Greenwich). 2018;20:1084–8.
2. Myers MG, Asmar R, Staessen JA. Office blood pressure measurement n the 21st century. J Clin Hypertens. 2018;20:1104–7.
3. O'Brien E, White WB, Parati G, Dolan E. Ambulatory blood pressure monitoring in the 21st century. J Clin Hypertens. 2018;20:1108–11.
4. Stergiou GS, Kario K, Kollias A, McManus RJ, Ohkubo T, Parati G, Imai Y. Home blood pressure monitoring in the 21st century. J Clin Hypertens. 2018;20:1116–21.
5. Stergiou G, Kollias A, Parati G, O'Brien E. Office blood pressure measurement: the weak cornerstone of hypertension diagnosis. Hypertension. 2018;71:813–5.
6. O'Brien E, Kario K, Staessen JA, de la Sierra A, Ohkubo T. Patterns of ambulatory blood pressure: clinical relevance and application. J Clin Hypertens (Greenwich). 2018;20:1112–5.
7. O'Brien E, Stergiou GS, Turner MJ. The quest for accuracy of blood pressure measuring devices. J Clin Hypertens (Greenwich). 2018;20:1093–5.

8. Whelton PK, Carey RM, Aronow WS, et al. ACC/AHA/AAPA/ABC/ACPM/AGS/APhA/ ASH/ASPC/NMA/PCNA Guideline for the prevention, detection, evaluation, and management of high blood pressure in adults: executive summary: a Report of the American College of Cardiology/American Heart Association Task Force on Clinical Practice Guidelines. Hypertension. 2018;71:e13–e115.

9. Pickering TG, James GD, Boddie C, Harshfield GA, Blank S, Laragh JH. How common is white coat hypertension? JAMA. 1988;259:225–8.

10. Owens P, Atkins N, O'Brien E. Diagnosis of White Coat Hypertension by Ambulatory Blood Pressure Monitoring. Hypertension. 1999;34:267–72.

11. O'Brien E, Parati G, Stergiou G, Asmar R, Beilin L, Bilo G, Clement D, de la Sierra A, de Leeuw P, Dolan E, Fagard R, Graves J, Head GA, Imai Y, Kario K, Lurbe E, Mallion JM, Mancia G, Mengden T, Myers M, Ogedegbe G, Ohkubo T, Omboni S, Palatini P, Redon J, Ruilope LM, Shennan A, Staessen JA, van Montfrans G, Verdecchia P, Waeber B, Wang J, Zanchetti A, Zhang Y, et al. European Society of Hypertension position paper on ambulatory blood pressure monitoring. J Hypertens. 2013;31:1731–68.

12. Anstey DE, Muntner P, Bello NA, Pugliese DN, Yano Y, Kronish IM, Reynolds K, Schwartz JE, Shimbo D. Diagnosing masked hypertension using ambulatory blood pressure monitoring, home blood pressure monitoring, or both? Hypertension. 2018;72:1200–7.

13. Pierdomenico SD, Pierdomenico AM, Coccina F, Clement DL, De Buyzere ML, De Bacquer DA, Ben-Dov IZ, Vongpatanasin W, Banegas JR, Ruilope LM, Thijs L, Staessen JA. Prognostic value of masked uncontrolled hypertension. Hypertension. 2018;72:862–9.

14. Staessen JA, Li Y, Hara A, Asayama K, Dolan E, O'Brien E. Blood pressure measurement anno 2016. Am J Hypertens. 2017;30:453–63.

15. Dolan E, O'Brien E. How should ambulatory blood pressure measurement be used in general practice? J Clin Hypertens (Greenwich). 2017;19:218–20.

16. Banegas JR, de la Cruz JJ, Graciani A, López-García E, Gijón-Conde T, Ruilope LM, Rodriguez-Artalejo F. Impact of ambulatory blood pressure monitoring on reclassification of hypertension prevalence and control in older people in Spain. J Clin Hypertens. 2015;17:453–61.

17. Salles GF, Reboldi G, Fagard RH, Cardoso CR, Pierdomenico SD, Verdecchia P, Eguchi K, Kario K, Hoshide S, Polonia J, de la Sierra A, Hermida RC, Dolan E, O'Brien E, Roush GC. Prognostic effect of the nocturnal blood pressure fall in hypertensive patients: the ambulatory blood pressure collaboration in patients with hypertension (ABC-H) meta-analysis. Hypertension. 2016;67:693–700.

18. Kollias A, Ntineri A, Stergiou GS. Association of night-time home blood pressure with night-time ambulatory blood pressure and target organ damage: a systematic review and meta-analysis. J Hypertens. 2017;35:442–52.

19. Parati G, Ochoa JE, Lombardi C, Bilo G. Assessment and management of blood pressure variability. Nat Rev Cardiol. 2013;10:143–55.

20. Stevens SL, Wood S, Koshiaris C, Law K, Glasziou P, Stevens RJ, McManus RJ. Blood pressure variability and cardiovascular disease: systematic review and meta-analysis. BMJ. 2016;354:i4098.

21. Parati G, Lombardi C, Hedner J, Bonsignore MR, Grote L, Tkacova R, Levy P, Riha R, Bassetti C, Narkiewicz K, Mancia G, McNicholas WT, European Respiratory Society; EU COST ACTION B26 members. Position paper on the management of patients with obstructive sleep apnea and hypertension: joint recommendations by the European Society of Hypertension, by the European Respiratory Society and by the members of European COST (COoperation in Scientific and Technological research) ACTION B26 on obstructive sleep apnea. J Hypertens. 2012;30:633–46.

22. Benetos A, Bulpitt CJ, Petrovic M, Ungar A, Agabiti Rosei E, Cherubini A, Redon J, Grodzicki T, Dominiczak A, Strandberg T, Mancia G. An Expert Opinion From the European Society of Hypertension-European Union Geriatric Medicine Society Working Group on the Management of Hypertension in Very Old, Frail Subjects. Hypertension. 2016;67:820–5.

23. O'Brien E, Dolan E. Ambulatory blood pressure measurement in the elderly: an opportunity to screen for atrial fibrillation. Hypertension. 2019;73:961–4.

24. Parati G, Dolan E, McManus RJ, Omboni S. Home blood pressure telemonitoring in the 21st century. J Clin Hypertens (Greenwich). 2018;20:1128–32.
25. Parati G, Stergiou GS, Asmar R, Bilo G, de Leeuw P, Imai Y, Kario K, Lurbe E, Manolis A, Mengden T, O'Brien E, Ohkubo T, Padfield P, Palatini P, Pickering T, Redon J, Revera M, Ruilope LM, Shennan A, Staessen JA, Tisler A, Waeber B, Zanchetti A, Mancia G. European Society of Hypertension guidelines for blood pressure monitoring at home: a summary report of the Second International Consensus Conference on Home Blood Pressure Monitoring. J Hypertens. 2008;26:1505–26.
26. Parati G, Stergiou GS, Asmar R, Bilo G, de Leeuw P, Imai Y, Kario K, Lurbe E, Manolis A, Mengden T, O'Brien E, Ohkubo T, Padfield P, Palatini P, Pickering TG, Redon J, Revera M, Ruilope LM, Shennan A, Staessen JA, Tisler A, Waeber B, Zanchetti A, Mancia G. European Society of Hypertension practice guidelines for home blood pressure monitoring. J Hum Hypertens. 2010;24:779–85.
27. Stergiou GS, Siontis KC, Ioannidis JP. Home blood pressure as a cardiovascular outcome predictor: it's time to take this method seriously. Hypertension. 2010;55:1301–3.
28. Stergiou GS, Asayama K, Thijs L, Kollias A, Niiranen TJ, Hozawa A, Boggia J, Johansson JK, Ohkubo T, Tsuji I, Jula AM, Imai Y, Staessen JA. Prognosis of white-coat and masked hypertension: International Database of HOme blood pressure in relation to Cardiovascular Outcome. Hypertension. 2014;63:675–82.
29. Ntineri A, Kalogeropoulos PG, Kyriakoulis KG, Aissopou EK, Thomopoulou G, Kollias A, Stergiou GS. Prognostic value of average home blood pressure and variability:19-year follow-up of the Didima study. J Hypertens. 2018;36:69–76.
30. Stergiou GS, Karpettas N, Destounis A, Tzamouranis D, Nasothimiou E, Kollias A, Roussias L, Moyssakis I. Home blood pressure monitoring alone vs. combined clinic and ambulatory measurements in following treatment-induced changes in blood pressure and organ damage. Am J Hypertens. 2014;27:184–92.
31. Agarwal R, Bills JE, Hecht TJ, Light RP. Role of home blood pressure monitoring in overcoming therapeutic inertia and improving hypertension control: a systematic review and meta-analysis. Hypertension. 2011;57:29–38.
32. McManus RJ, Mant J, Franssen M, et al. Telemonitoring and/or self-monitoring of blood pressure in hypertension (TASMINH4): A Randomised Controlled Trial. J Hypertens. 2018;36:e5.
33. Asayama K, Ohkubo T, Metoki H, Obara T, Inoue R, Kikuya M, Thijs L, Staessen JA, Imai Y. Cardiovascular outcomes in the first trial of antihypertensive therapy guided by self-measured home blood pressure. Hypertens Res. 2012;35:1102–10.
34. Verberk WJ, Omboni S, Kollias A, Stergiou GS. Screening for atrial fibrillation with automated blood pressure measurement: Research evidence and practice recommendations. Int J Cardiol. 2016;203:465–73.
35. Parati G, Omboni S, Albini F, Piantoni L, Giuliano A, Revera M, Illyes M, Mancia G. Home blood pressure telemonitoring improves hypertension control in general practice. The TeleBPCare study. J Hypertens. 2009;27:198–203.

Guidelines for Home Blood Pressure Monitoring

16

George S. Stergiou, Gianfranco Parati, Yutaka Imai,
Richard J. McManus, Geoff A. Head, Kazuomi Kario,
Paul Muntner, Martin G. Myers, James Sharman,
Eoin O'Brien, Michael A. Weber, Paul K. Whelton,
and Giuseppe Mancia

G. S. Stergiou (✉)
Hypertension Center STRIDE-7, National and Kapodistrian University of Athens, School of
Medicine, Third Department of Medicine, Sotiria Hospital, Athens, Greece
e-mail: gstergi@med.uoa.gr

G. Parati
Department of Medicine and Surgery, University of Milano-Bicocca, Milan, Italy

Istituto Auxologico Italiano, IRCCS, Department of Cardiovascular, Neural and Metabolic
Sciences, Milan, Italy
e-mail: gianfranco.parati@unimib.it

Y. Imai
Tohoku Institute for Management of Blood Pressure, Sendai, Japan
e-mail: yutaka.imai.d6@tohoku.ac.jp

R. J. McManus
Nuffield Department of Primary Care Health Sciences, University of Oxford,
Radcliffe Observatory Quarter, Oxford, UK
e-mail: richard.mcmanus@phc.ox.ac.uk

G. A. Head
Baker Heart and Diabetes Institute, Melbourne, VIC, Australia
e-mail: Geoff.Head@baker.edu.au

K. Kario
Division of Cardiovascular Medicine, Department of Medicine, Jichi Medical University
School of Medicine (JMU), Tochigi, Japan
e-mail: kkario@jichi.ac.jp

P. Muntner
Department of Epidemiology, University of Alabama at Birmingham, Birmingham, AL, USA
e-mail: pmuntner@uab.edu

M. G. Myers
Division of Cardiology, Schulich Heart Program, Sunnybrook Health Sciences Centre,
Toronto, ON, Canada

Department of Medicine, University of Toronto, Toronto, ON, Canada
e-mail: martin.myers@sunnybrook.ca

J. Sharman
Menzies Institute for Medical Research, University of Tasmania, Hobart, TAS, Australia
e-mail: james.sharman@utas.edu.au

E. O'Brien
The Conway Institute, University College Dublin, Dublin, Ireland

M. A. Weber
Division of Cardiovascular Medicine, State University of New York, Downstate Medical
Center, New York, NY, USA

P. K. Whelton
Department of Epidemiology, Tulane University School of Public Health and Tropical
Medicine, New Orleans, LA, USA

Department of Medicine, Tulane University School of Medicine, New Orleans, LA, USA

G. Mancia
University of Milano-Bicocca, Milan, Italy
e-mail: giuseppe.mancia@unimib.it

For more than three decades, guidelines presented by some scientific societies around the world have recommended home blood pressure monitoring (HBPM) for patients with hypertension [1, 2]. However, others have hesitated, probably because published evidence on the clinical application of HBPM and outcome studies have been reported much later than for ambulatory blood pressure monitoring (ABPM) [3, 4]. The publication of several outcome studies during the last 20 years reporting the superiority of HBPM compared to office blood pressure has now supported a major role for HBPM in hypertension decision-making [3–7].

Many patients with hypertension around the world have long ago chosen to use the method for self-monitoring their blood pressure at home with costs absorbed by themselves [8, 9]. The manufacturing industry has responded to this market demand and opportunity by releasing a wide variety of low-cost devices for self-HBPM into the market. Initially, most HBPM devices were auscultatory (mostly aneroid), whereas currently most are automated oscillometric. This "consumer oriented" development of HBPM devices has not always fulfilled the rigorous standards for measurement accuracy demanded by science, which is necessary for making important diagnostic and treatment decisions (www.stridebp.org) [10, 11].

Statements and guidelines for using HBPM which have been developed by scientific organizations around the world during the last three decades are presented in Table 16.1 [2, 3, 9, 12–24]. An algorithm for using HBPM was first presented by Thomas Pickering in his 1990 book on "*Ambulatory monitoring and blood pressure variability*" [1]. In 1995, the American Society of Hypertension was the first organization to recommend an algorithm for diagnosing hypertension with HBPM, which however required confirmation by ABPM [2].

Table 16.1 Guidelines by scientific societies for home blood pressure monitoring

Body	Year	Recommendation on main indications for clinical use
ASH [2]	1995	Confirm elevated office BP by HBPM. If they disagree confirm by ABPM
CHS [12]	1999	When HBPM is used to assess WCH, the latter should be confirmed by ABPM if available
Australia [13]	1999	Vague recommendations for detecting and following WCH and the treatment effects
FSH [14]	2000	HBPM could be used for screening subjects with office hypertension, but if low ABPM is required. Seems appropriate for following WCH
ESH [15]	2003	Unclear recommendation for detecting and following WCH
JSH [16]	2003	HBPM suitable for the diagnosis of intractable hypertension and WCH and to assess treatment effects
ESH [17]	2004	Can be used as screening method for WCH but requires confirmation by ABPM
AHA [18]	2005	HBPM can be used for initial diagnosis and treatment evaluation
ASH [19]	2008	Use HBPM to confirm office hypertension: If low continue to monitor; if high treat; if borderline confirm by ABPM
ESH [3, 20]	2008 2010	HBPM to be used by all treated hypertensives and to detect WCH and MH. If disagrees with ABPM, the latter should probably take precedence
AHA, ASH [21]	2008	HBPM should be reimbursed and routinely used in most patients with known or suspected hypertension. Confirm office hypertension by HBPM: if low continue to monitor; if high treat; if borderline confirm by ABPM
JSH [9]	2012	HBPM is essential for the diagnosis of WCH and MH and extremely effective for the evaluation of drug effects and facilitates long-term BP control
USPSTF [22]	2015	HBPM may be acceptable for confining hypertension (ABPM preferred)
Australia [23]	2015	HBPM can be used to detect WCH and MH and to estimate the effectiveness of treatment
HOPE Asia [24]	2018	Base diagnoses on office BP and HBPM. When they disagree give priority to HBPM and if possible confirm by ABPM

ABPM ambulatory blood pressure monitoring, *ACC* American College of Cardiology, *AHA* American Heart Association, *ASH* American Society of Hypertension, *CHS* Canadian Hypertension Society, *ESC* European Society of Cardiology, *ESH* European Society of Hypertension, *FSH* French Society of Hypertension, *HBPM* home blood pressure monitoring, *HOPE Asia Network* Hypertension Cardiovascular Outcome Prevention and Evidence in Asia, *JSH* Japanese Society of Hypertension, *MH* masked hypertension, *WCH* white coat hypertension

In 1999, the Canadian Hypertension Society adopted a similar approach for the use of HBPM [12], and in 2005 the Canadian Hypertension Education Program included HBPM in their recommended algorithm for the diagnosis of hypertension [25]. In 2006, the UK National Institute for Health and Clinical Excellence (NICE) guidelines for management of hypertension stated that HBPM and ABPM should not be used because their value had not been adequately established and further research was necessary (*partial update of NICE clinical guideline 18, June 2006*). However, in 2011 the NICE made the landmark recommendation that ABPM is necessary to confirm the diagnosis of hypertension in subjects with office hypertension at stages 1–2, but indicated that HBPM was a *suitable alternative* in those unable to tolerate ABPM [26]. Meanwhile, other organizations such as the European Society of Hypertension (ESH) [3, 15, 17], the American Heart Association [18], the American Society of Hypertension [19], the French Society of Hypertension [14], the Japanese Society of Hypertension [9, 16], and Australian organizations [13, 23] published scientific statements and guidelines specific for HBPM, in which this method was strongly supported for a major role in the diagnosis and management of hypertension (Table 16.1). In 2008, Thomas Pickering led a joint scientific statement by the American Heart Association and the American Society of Hypertension calling for the wide use of HBPM in most subjects with suspected or treated hypertension and recommended reimbursement for the method [21]. In the same year the ESH Working Group on Blood Pressure Monitoring also published HBPM guidelines which were very much in line with the American ones [3, 21, 27].

The 2017 American College of Cardiology/American Heart Association blood pressure guidelines [6] and the 2018 guidelines by the European Society of Cardiology/European Society of Hypertension [7] highlighted the role of HBPM as well as ABPM in the diagnosis and management of hypertension and started a new era in hypertension management on both sides of the Atlantic by endorsing out-of-office blood pressure measurement as mandatory for most diagnostic and treatment decisions (Table 16.2). However, the European guidelines still gave the option of basing the diagnosis of hypertension on repeated office blood pressure measurements taken on several visits, which probably presents a realistic approach given the limitations in the availability of HBPM and especially for ABPM [7].

ABPM has some advantages compared with HBPM, including (a) stronger published clinical outcome evidence, (b) measurements that are fully automated and thereby unbiased (no observers involved in the measurement process and reporting of readings), (c) the capacity to evaluate blood pressure at work and during sleep, and (d) results that are automatically summarized and available within 24 h [4]. Although the current technology of HBPM devices can accommodate unbiased reporting of measurements (automated memory, PC link, or telemonitoring) and also automated nocturnal measurements during sleep, these are rarely obtained in clinical practice [3]. This may be why most scientific societies recommend ABPM as the "primary method" for hypertension diagnosis with HBPM being a "useful alterative" (Table 16.1). However, HBPM is much more widely available than ABPM and is preferred by most patients and, therefore, it is more appropriate for repeated and long-term use [3, 4, 28]. Thus, a pragmatic approach for most scientific societies and healthcare organizations is to promote HBPM as much as ABPM,

Table 16.2 Recommendations for using home blood pressure monitoring in the latest American and European guidelines for the management of hypertension

| ACC/ AHA [6] | 2017 | Use ABPM or HBPM: in office BP 120–160/80–100 mmHg to detect WCH and MH; to confirm the diagnosis of hypertension; for treatment titration |
| ESC/ESH [7] | 2018 | Use ABPM or HBPM in most adults with office BP 130–159/85–99 mmHg to detect WCH and MH and other indications |

ACC American College of Cardiology, *AHA* American Heart Association, *ESC* European Society of Cardiology, *ESH* European Society of Hypertension, *ABPM* ambulatory blood pressure monitoring, *HBPM* home blood pressure monitoring, *MH* masked hypertension, *WCH* white coat hypertension

aiming to increase the number of people having their blood pressure status confirmed by out-of-office readings (Table 16.1).

In conclusion, considerable evidence regarding the clinical utility of HBPM has been accumulated during the last three decades. This has resulted in scientific societies recommending HBPM as an important source of information for the evaluation and management of adults with suspected or treated hypertension. The most recent guidelines are in agreement that the use of HBPM is important to optimize the management of hypertension in clinical practice. Additional efforts to implement the use of HBPM would likely enhance the diagnosis and control of hypertension across communities.

References

1. Pickering TG. Self-monitoring of blood pressure. In: Ambulatory monitoring and blood pressure variability (Part 1). London: Science Press; 1991. p. 8.5.
2. Pickering TG. Recommendations for the use of home (self) and ambulatory blood pressure monitoring. American Society of Hypertension Ad Hoc Panel. Am J Hypertens. 1996;9:1–11.
3. Parati G, Stergiou GS, Asmar R, Bilo G, de Leeuw P, Imai Y, et al. European Society of Hypertension guidelines for blood pressure monitoring at home: a summary report of the Second International Consensus Conference on Home Blood Pressure Monitoring. J Hypertens. 2008;26:1505–26.
4. O'Brien E, Parati G, Stergiou G, Asmar R, Beilin L, Bilo G, et al. European Society of Hypertension position paper on ambulatory blood pressure monitoring. J Hypertens. 2013;31:1731–68.
5. Stergiou GS, Asayama K, Thijs L, Kollias A, Niiranen TJ, Hozawa A, et al. Prognosis of white-coat and masked hypertension: International Database of HOme blood pressure in relation to Cardiovascular Outcome. Hypertension. 2014;63(4):675–82.
6. Whelton PK, Carey RM, Aronow WS, Casey DE Jr, Collins KJ, Dennison Himmelfarb C, et al. 2017 ACC/AHA/AAPA/ABC/ACPM/AGS/APhA/ASH/ASPC/NMA/PCNA guideline for the prevention, detection, evaluation and management of high blood pressure in adults: a report of the American College of Cardiology/American Heart Association Task Force on clinical practice guidelines. Hypertension. 2018;71:e13–e115.
7. Williams B, Mancia G, Spiering W, Agabiti Rosei E, Azizi M, Burnier M, et al. 2018 ESC/ESH Guidelines for the management of arterial hypertension: The Task Force for the management of arterial hypertension of the European Society of Cardiology and the European Society of Hypertension. J Hypertens. 2018;36:1953–2041.
8. Tsakiri C, Stergiou GS, Boivin JM. Implementation of home blood pressure monitoring in clinical practice. Clin Exp Hypertens. 2013;35:558–62.
9. Imai Y, Kario K, Shimada K, Kawano Y, Hasebe N, Matsuura H, et al. The Japanese Society of Hypertension Guidelines for Self-monitoring of Blood Pressure at Home (Second Edition). Hypertens Res. 2012;35:777–95.
10. Jung MH, Kim GH, Kim JH, Moon KW, Yoo KD, Rho TH, et al. Reliability of home blood pressure monitoring: in the context of validation and accuracy. Blood Press Monit. 2015;20:215–20.
11. Akpolat T, Dilek M, Aydogdu T, Adibelli Z, Erdem DG, Erdem E. Home sphygmomanometers: validation versus accuracy. Blood Press Monit. 2009;14:26–31.
12. Myers MG, Haynes RB, Rabkin SW. Canadian hypertension society guidelines for ambulatory blood pressure monitoring. Am J Hypertens. 1999;12:1149–57.
13. Stowasser M, Armstrong R. Self-measurement of blood pressure: a paper for health professionals. National Heart Foundation of Australia 1999. www.heartfoundation.com.au. Accessed 18 Dec 2018.

14. Asmar R, Zanchetti A. Guidelines for the use of self-blood pressure monitoring: a summary report of the First International Consensus Conference. Groupe Evaluation & Measure of the French Society of Hypertension. J Hypertens. 2000;18:493–508.
15. O'Brien E, Asmar R, Beilin L, Imai Y, Mallion JM, Mancia G, et al. European Society of Hypertension recommendations for conventional, ambulatory and home blood pressure measurement. J Hypertens. 2003;21:821–48.
16. Imai Y, Otsuka K, Kawano Y, Shimada K, Hayashi H, Tochikubo O, et al. Japanese Society of Hypertension (JSH) guidelines for self-monitoring of blood pressure at home. Hypertens Res. 2003;26:771–82.
17. Stergiou G, Mengden T, Padfield PL, Parati G, O'Brien E. Working Group on Blood Pressure Monitoring of the European Society of Hypertension. Self monitoring of blood pressure at home. BMJ. 2004;329:870–1.
18. Pickering TG, Hall JE, Appel LJ, Falkner BE, Graves J, Hill MN, et al. Recommendations for blood pressure measurement in humans and experimental animals. Part 1. Blood pressure measurement in humans: a statement for professionals from the Subcommittee of Professional and Public Education of the American Heart Association Council on High Blood Pressure Research. Hypertension. 2005;45:142–61.
19. Pickering TG, White WB, American Society of Hypertension Writing Group. American Society of Hypertension Position Paper: when and how to use self (home) and ambulatory blood pressure monitoring. J Clin Hypertens. 2008;10:850–5.
20. Parati G, Stergiou GS, Asmar R, Bilo G, de Leeuw P, Imai Y, et al. European Society of Hypertension practice guidelines for home blood pressure monitoring. J Hum Hypertens. 2010;24:779–85.
21. Pickering TG, Miller NH, Ogedegbe G, Krakoff LR, Artinian NT, Goff D, et al. Call to action on use and reimbursement for home blood pressure monitoring: executive summary: a joint scientific statement from the American Heart Association, American Society of Hypertension, and Preventive Cardiovascular Nurses Association. Hypertension. 2008;52:1–9.
22. Siu AL, Preventive Services Task Force US. Screening for high blood pressure in adults: U.S. Preventive Services Task Force recommendation statement. Ann Intern Med. 2015;163(10):778–86.
23. Sharman JE, Howes FS, Head GA, et al. Home blood pressure monitoring: Australian expert consensus statement. J Hypertens. 2015;33:1721–8.
24. Park S, Buranakitjaroen P, Chen CH, Chia YC, Divinagracia R, Hoshide S, et al. Expert panel consensus recommendations for home blood pressure monitoring in Asia: the Hope Asia Network. J Hum Hypertens. 2018;32:249–58.
25. Myers MG, Tobe SW, McKay DW, Bolli P, Hemmelgarn BR, McAlister FA, et al. New algorithm for the diagnosis of hypertension. Am J Hypertens. 2005;18:1369–74.
26. National Institute for Health and Clinical Excellence (NICE). Hypertension: the clinical management of primary hypertension in adults. Clinical Guideline. 2011;127. www.nice.org.uk/guidance/CG127. Accessed 18 Dec 2018
27. Parati G, Pickering TG. Home blood-pressure monitoring: US and European consensus. Lancet. 2009;373(9667):876–8.
28. Wood S, Greenfield SM, Sayeed Haque M, Martin U, Gill PS, Mant J, et al. Influence of ethnicity on acceptability of method of blood pressure monitoring: a cross-sectional study in primary care. Br J Gen Pract. 2016;66:e577–86.

Index

© The Editor(s), under exclusive license to Springer Nature Switzerland AG 2020
G. S. Stergiou et al. (eds.), *Home Blood Pressure Monitoring*,
Updates in Hypertension and Cardiovascular Protection,
https://doi.org/10.1007/978-3-030-23065-4

The manufacturer's authorised representative in the EU is Springer
Nature Customer Service Centre GmbH, Europaplatz 3, 69115 Heidelberg,
Germany. If you have any concerns regarding our products, please
contact ProductSafety@springernature.com

Printed and bound by CPI Group (UK) Ltd, Croydon, CR0 4YY
29/04/2026
02099715-0001